Navigating the Complexities of Health Professions Education for Millennial and Generation Z Learners

GENERATIONAL DIFFERENCES IN HIGHER EDUCATION AND THE WORKPLACE: LEADING AND TEACHING MILLENNIALS AND GENERATION Z

Series Editor: Michael G. Strawser, University of Central Florida, and Deanna Sellnow, University of Central Florida

Members of Generation Z, the post-millennial generation, are independent, entrepreneurial and technologically engaged. Gen Z, otherwise known as the iGeneration, value loyalty, consider themselves to be open-minded and compassionate, and their digital literacy is unprecedented. While higher education institutions have been evolving to meet the needs of Millennials, Generation Z students have quietly become the traditional higher ed. consumer. As the largest population cohort, edging out both the millennials and the Boomers, "Z" should be a subject ripe for education inquiry, especially in higher ed. settings and, as "Z" members transition to the workforce, the corporate setting. Thus, this interdisciplinary series examines the intersection of higher education and unique generational variances. This series is receptive to works that use a variety of methodological approaches, focus on any recent generational dynamics, and situate their analysis in higher education and corporate contexts. Generational Differences in Higher Education and the Workplace: Leading and Teaching Millennials and Generation Z seeks to be truly interdisciplinary by including authors from all the social sciences and humanities: communication, history, sociology, economics, philosophy, psychology, ethics, as well as education and business.

Recent Titles in This Series

Navigating the Complexities of Health Professions Education for Millennial and Generation Z Learners
By Channing R. Ford, Kimberly B. Garza, Lindsey E. Moseley, and Emily B. Wilkins

The COVID-19 Impact on Higher Education Stakeholders and Institutional Services
Edited by Michael G. Strawser

Higher Education Implications for Teaching and Learning during COVID-19
Edited by Michael G. Strawser

The COVID-19 Impact on Higher Education Stakeholders and Institutional Services
Edited by Michael G. Strawser

Leading Millennial Faculty: Navigating the New Professorate
Edited by Michael G. Strawser

Recruitment, Retention, and Engagement of a Millennial Workforce
Edited by Stephanie A. Smith

Navigating the Complexities of Health Professions Education for Millennial and Generation Z Learners

Channing R. Ford, Kimberly B. Garza,
Lindsey E. Moseley,
and Emily B. Wilkins

LEXINGTON BOOKS
Lanham • Boulder • New York • London

Published by Lexington Books
An imprint of The Rowman & Littlefield Publishing Group, Inc.
4501 Forbes Boulevard, Suite 200, Lanham, Maryland 20706
www.rowman.com

86-90 Paul Street, London EC2A 4NE

British Library Cataloguing in Publication Information Available

Library of Congress Cataloging-in-Publication Data

Library of Congress Cataloging-in-Publication DataNames: Ford, Channing R., author. | Garza, Kimberly, 1975- author. | Moseley, Lindsey E., author. | Wilkins, Emily B., author.
Title: Navigating the complexities of health professions education for Millennial and Generation Z learners / Channing R. Ford, Kimberly B. Garza, Lindsey E. Moseley, and Emily B. Wilkins.
Description: Lanham : Lexington Books, [2024] | Series: Generational differences in higher education and the workplace: leading and teaching Millennials and Generation Z | Includes bibliographical references and index.
Identifiers: LCCN 2023049750 (print) | LCCN 2023049751 (ebook) | ISBN 9781666917895 (cloth) | ISBN 9781666917901 (epub)
Subjects: LCSH: Medical education--United States. | Generation Y--Education (Higher)--United States. | Generation Z--Education (Higher)--United States. | Student-centered learning--United States.
Classification: LCC R745 .F67 2024 (print) | LCC R745 (ebook) | DDC 610.71--dc23/eng/20231214
LC record available at https://lccn.loc.gov/2023049750
LC ebook record available at https://lccn.loc.gov/2023049751

Contents

Acknowledgments

The authors would like to acknowledge Dr. Kristen Helms for her time and efforts in supporting the revision of this book.

Preface

The goal of this book is to offer new insights into the complexities of teaching and training the modern generations of students. More specifically, the book explores nuanced topics that are relevant to Generation Z learners and their predecessors, the Millennials. These generations were chosen as the centerpiece because they comprise the current student population in higher education at the time of this book.

The context of this generational exploration is within health professions education. Thus, the audience for this book is largely health professions educators, which includes anyone on a college or university campus who influences student development inside or outside the learning environment. This consists of college faculty, clinical preceptors, institutional administrators, and university staff. Further, while the book was written with educators in mind, it was specifically aimed at ones who are of prior generations (i.e., Gen X or Baby Boomers), or those who might be unsure how to cultivate the best learning environments for their Millennial or Gen Z students.

Health professions education encompasses many health-related disciplines. While the book is peppered with an assortment of examples from different health professions, the authors' goal was not to offer a comprehensive view of all disciplines in all instances. Rather, examples of different health professions were threaded throughout if a topic was specifically relevant to a discipline or if examples from different fields helped to exemplify a specific point the authors were making. Additionally, authors utilized the data and studies that were accessible.

This book was written in a scholarly manner, with the inclusion of national data sets and research studies that, when synthesized, built a credible body of chapters. The inclusion of web-based articles, blogs, and commentaries helped the authors make relevant points or summarize key findings. The authors explored the topics in the chapters based on work from the foremost experts in the fields. A comprehensive list of references is available at the end of the book.

While the book offers a deep dive into generational theory and a comparison of Millennials and Generation Z on an assortment of topics, the authors hope that healthcare educators glean practical insights as well. Recommendations for cultivating a positive learning environment are available throughout the chapters, with a balanced view of topics inside and outside the classroom. To this end, while the book offers insights and explanations on Millennials and Generation Z within health professions, the authors hope that it continues the conversation on the dynamic, and often challenging enterprise of being a contemporary college or university educator.

Chapter 1

Overview of Generational Theory and the Millennial Generation

Traversing the educational landscape of higher education continues to challenge educators with the constantly evolving expectations of learners. "Since the days of the Old Testament and ancient Greece, the word 'generation' and its various roots have connected the essence of life-birth and death, the maturing of youth and the letting-go of old age, the rise and fall of dynasties and nations" (Strauss and Howe 1991, 59). Strauss and Howe's quote speaks to the role each generation plays in the revitalization and reinvention of society. Furthermore, they stress within their text, the need to better understand each generation in order to adapt the learning environment to support learners' development. Essentially, it is time to embrace what makes every generation unique and what drives them (Gerhardt, Nachemson-Ekwall, and Fogel 2021). Historically, educators have relied on standard teaching and learning practices to prepare students for the next step of their academic journey. The adage "sage on the stage" was one such approach that faculty gravitated toward as it provided a sense of security by limiting the need for student engagement. Yet, now, this approach is considered outdated and spurned for the distance it places between educator and learner.

Adopting proven instructional practices that are focused on student engagement is essential for today's learning environments. Engaging students using traditional learning approaches is not enough. Continued professional development is required to ensure that faculty are prepared to develop mentoring relationships that meet the learners' expectations. Furthermore, educators must understand how these expectations differ by student, by generation, and by region. As these expectations are driven by learners, faculty must be aware of what those expectations are, and how to adapt and adopt the learning strategies that will best serve students. This chapter will examine the role of generational theory, provide a brief overview of previous generational traits, and an examination of the Millennial Generation.

GENERATIONAL THEORY

Recognizing and understanding how learners' expectations change over time will ensure that educators are prepared for a diverse and dynamic learning environment. A generational identity is not intended to assign a label as it is simply one of the elements that influences an individual's identity. "Fundamentally, generations were invented as a way to categorize and help us better understand the phenomenon and impact of broad age differences" (Gerhardt, Nachemson-Ekwall, and Fogel 2021, 24). Essentially, generational identity should be considered as one element of an individual and serve as a lens that helps one understand differences. The role of generational theory in academia is well-established and has allowed scholars and educators to examine how characteristics and expectations shape each new cohort of learners as they enter the classroom. Kupperschmidt defines a generation as "a group of people or cohorts who share birth years and experiences as they move through time together, influencing and being influenced by a variety of critical factors" (2000, 66).

Strauss and Howe, often considered the authority on generational modeling (Coomes and DeBard 2004), define generations as "a cohort-group whose length approximates the span of a phase of life and whose boundaries are fixed by peer personality" (Strauss and Howe 1991). A peer personality encompasses the evolution of behavioral traits and attitudes the generation portrays across the trajectory of its lifecycle. Within Strauss and Howe's (1991) model, each phase of life results in a new manifestation with each phase typically lasting around 22 years. The phases are known as youth (0–21 years), rising adulthood (22–43 years), midlife (44–65 years), and elderhood (66–87 years). These phases were defined as stages of dependence (youth), activity (rising adulthood), leadership (midlife), and stewardship (elderhood).

These lifecycle generations have shown that each generational peer personality expresses itself differently as they move from one phase to the next. Strauss and Howe illustrate that each generation has a peer personality, which they define as a "generational persona recognized and determined by (1) common age location; (2) common beliefs and behaviors; and (3) perceived membership in a common generation" (1991, 64). They note that the most important element of the generation's peer personality is its ability to recognize how it differs from other generations and what makes that generation its own. In their later work, Howe and Strauss (2000) refer to peer personality as generational persona and defined it as being distinctly and variably human, and embodying attitudes regarding all aspects of life including culture, home life, institutions, lifestyles, politics, religion, and their own future.

Within their model, Strauss and Howe (1991) propose four generational types (idealist, reactive, civic, and adaptive) that are characterized as dominant or recessive. They note the flow between generations stating, "During a spiritual awakening, Idealists are moving into rising adulthood while Reactives are appearing as children; during a secular crisis, Civics are moving into rising adulthood while Adaptives are appearing as children" (Strauss and Howe, 1991, 35). Each generational type evolves with each new monumental event, spurring the next cohort to enter the next development phase. Furthermore, at a later point in time, this same generation triggers a different social moment, which results in the cycle beginning again.

These four generational types each display their own unique traits. Idealists pick apart established institutions implemented by older generations prior to retreating into a self-absorbed stasis; later as they mature, they navigate toward uncompromising moralists. Reactives are the risk takers, spending most of their 20s fighting the good fight only to mellow as they become older adults. Civics create the establishment, serving as the aggressive founders of institutions and continue to defend those institutions as they age. Lastly, adaptives are "elder-focused conformists early in life, but junior-focused pluralists later on" (Strauss and Howe 1991, 39).

How a Generational Cohort Evolves

In their earlier work, Howe and Strauss (2000) noted that each new generation follows three basic principles to redirect society: (1) solves a problem that impacted a prior generation; (2) corrects the current midlife generations behavioral excess; and (3) replaces the social role of the elder generation. Later in their book, *Millennials Go to College*, Howe and Strauss (2003) amend their earlier findings and redefine these three principles as how a generation rebels from those that came before them. They outline that each generation rebels in three ways: (1) they break away from the generation before them as they identify the previous generation's style no longer functions within the new era; (2) it rebels from the excessive nature of the midlife generation often as a mechanism of protest or with support from the midlife generation who recognizes their shortcomings; and (3) to fill the role the elderhood generation is vacating. These three basic rebellion tactics apply to any rising generation as it allows the younger generation the freedom to redefine their definition of what it means to be young and to direct society as they deem appropriate. Furthermore, Howe and Strauss (2003) identified three rules for navigating what they refer to as the generational diagonal which posits: (1) the new generation will break away from the generation proceeding them; (2) the new generation will address the errors of the generation currently at the midlife stage; and (3) the new generation will strive to fill the social roles being vacated by the elder generation. Coomes and DeBard (2004) examined Howe and Strauss's theory further to assess how it impacts a generational cohort's evolution. They propose that generations are not static and are influenced by historical events as they move through time.

However, it is important to recognize that not all members of a particular generational cohort will look the same; older cohort members can look very different from the younger cohort members of the same generational cohort. Older members may share similarities with the generation before them, while younger members may have similar qualities to the next generation (Seemiller and Grace 2019b). "Consequently, individuals born on the cusp of a generation may not see themselves in the typical narrative for their generation, perhaps finding more connection with the neighboring cohort" (Gerhardt, Nachemson-Ekwall, and Fogel 2021, 29). These members are described as "cuspers" and are known as micro-generations. The micro-generation between Generation X and older Millennials are known as Xennials and the micro-generation between Millennials and Generation Z are known as Zennials. These cuspers often portray generational traits from the generation prior to them as well as the current one.

While the commonality of birth year establishes the cohort, each generation is further influenced by environmental, sociocultural, and socioeconomic events that impact one's personality, values, beliefs, and expectations (Seemiller and Grace 2019b; Srinivasan 2012). Both sociocultural (war, new technology, familial changes) and socioeconomic events (job scarcity or security) can shape or reshape a generation with each new event. As the generation navigates each new life event, they develop characteristics that differentiate themselves from those in the generation before and after them. These differences are often reflected within their personalities, and how they approach work to include their attitude and what motivates them (Srinivasan 2012). Older generations can impact younger generations' societal views as the political decisions of the older generation shaped the world the younger generations are inhabiting (Seemiller and Grace 2019b). While themes and commonalities will always exist between generations, there will also be outliers. Each generation displays both positive and negative traits unique to them.

Researchers should also consider the lifecycle, cohort, and period effects of societal events when considering the length of a generation. The period effect pertains to one's response to experiencing an event, circumstance, or societal force (Seemiller and Grace 2019b). These events often have long-term effects that leave a lasting impression on the generation. Pop culture often aligns with a period effect.

The differences in how generational cohorts develop are known as a cohort effect. These differences are often the result of witnessing a historical or societal event. The level of influence is dependent on the age of the cohort, having a more dynamic impression when experienced during adolescence or young adulthood. Lastly, as a result of the dynamic landscape of today's 24-hour news cycle, technological advancements, and access to information at the push of a button, these generational cycles have shortened. Seemiller and Grace (2019b) postulate that generations now span between 14 and 20 years. Whereas, Gerhardt and colleagues (2021) propose that Traditional and Baby Boomer generations span 19 years, and Millennial and Generation Z generations span 16 years.

STUDENT DEMOGRAPHICS IN HIGHER EDUCATION

The National Center for Education Statistics' (NCES) data shows that in 2020, there were 15.9 million baccalaureate students and 3.1 million post-baccalaureate students enrolled in degree granting institutions (National Center for Education Statistics [NCES] 2022). In fall 2021, there were less baccalaureate students enrolled at just 15.4 million in U.S. degree granting institutions with a slight increase in enrollment at the post-baccalaureate level at 3.2 million. Of those in undergraduate degree programs, 70% were enrolled in 4-year institutions and 30% were enrolled in 2-year institutions. Of those enrolled in 4-year institutions, 73% were full-time students in comparison to 2-year institutions where 35% of students were enrolled full-time. When considering graduate students, 1.8 million (57%) were enrolled full-time and 1.4 million (43%) at part-time. (NCES 2022)

The age distribution of these populations varied at the differing academic levels; 91% of undergraduate students at 4-year public institutions were aged 25 years of age or younger. When considering this same age group at other types of institutions, 85% of undergraduates at private 4-year institutions in this same age category were enrolled and 79% at public 2-year institutions. Of those pursuing post-baccalaureate education, 66% of full-time enrollees were under thirty years of age in public and private nonprofit institutions. However, in for-profit institutions, these numbers differed with 66% of students aged 30 years of age or older. Lastly, when looking at part-time graduate students considering an age of thirty years or older, 78% of those enrolled at private for-profit institutions, 63% at private nonprofit institutions, and 59% at public institutions fit this age demographic (NCES 2022).

As the data shows, higher education is experiencing a decline in undergraduate enrollment as is to be expected with the approaching demographic cliff. However, increased enrollment in graduate education serves as a reminder that educators should be aware that student enrollment may differ within and across academic levels. Furthermore, educators should be cognizant of the needs of the varying generations within the learning environment and be prepared to adapt accordingly.

HISTORICAL LOOK AT PREVIOUS GENERATIONS

Before delving into the characteristics of the Millennial generation, it is important to have a broader understanding of the generations that came before them. A brief snapshot will be provided for the earlier cohorts to provide additional context as to how Millennials and Generation Z were influenced by the generations before them.

Lost Generation (1883–1900)

This generation grew up fast due to their socioeconomic circumstances. "As children, their violence, independence, and low educational achievement worried parents" (Howe and Strauss 2003, 19). This generation was responsible for a number of economic innovations including the advent of the supermarket, radio, and aviation. This generation navigated the Great Depression and World War II, and as they transitioned into their role as elders, they garnered a distrust of those in power and expected very little (Howe and Strauss 2003).

G.I. Generation (1901–1924)

Seen as "the good kids," this generation grew up in a period when going to school was on the rise and child labor was on the decline. They were actively involved in World War II and as recipients of the G.I. Bill, they used those opportunities to change the world around them. They helped establish the suburbs, pioneered the development of vaccines, and helped get society to the moon. As society elders, their influence on culture and societal values was limited. (Howe and Strauss 2003)

Silent Generation (1925–1942)

They were influenced by the Great Depression and World War II and as a result were referred to as children of "war and Depression" (Howe and Strauss 2003, 19). However, they missed being known as heroes of war and instead have been seen as risk averse. The Silent Generation are also known as the Traditionalists (Desy et al. 2017) and were considered to be hard working, obedient, and familiar with sacrifice. This generation was more concerned with keeping on the straight and narrow, than pushing against the tide. They "planned on early marriages and long careers with big organizations" (Howe and Strauss 2003, 12).

Baby Boomers (1943–1960)

While there are differences of opinion regarding the cohort years of this generation with Howe and Strauss (2003) supporting the year span articulated above and Gerhardt, Nachemson-Ekwall, and Fogel (2021) indicating the year span as 1946–1964, scholars describe the generation in a similar manner. They are seen as explorers, familiar with change, and known for questioning authority and the rules (Desy et al. 2017). Baby Boomers are a generation that came of age during a period of economic growth, and as a result focused on climbing the corporate ladder. Baby Boomers helped foster progressive shifts and participated in society events such as the March on Washington, Civil Rights, and so on (Howe and Strauss 2003). This generation coined the term "workaholic" establishing a 60–70 hour work week. Their role in the Women's Movement supported the adoption of the dual-career household as well as the single-parent household; while this diversity provided opportunities for women within the workforce, it also created issues with childcare.

Generation X (1961–1981)

This generation marked the first decrease in birth rates since 1946 (Gerhardt, Nachemson-Ekwall, and Fogel 2021). Known as a skeptical generation, they were born into a time of skepticism and caution. During this time, divorce rates doubled, working parents created latch-key children who were left to their own devices and grew up with limited parental influence. This resulted in a generation of independent and self-reliant individuals who wanted clear delineations between work life and home life. This distinct need for work–life balance marked a significant deviation from the Boomer and Traditional generations, with them often being referred to as the "slacker" generation by the older cohorts (Gerhardt, Nachemson-Ekwall, and Fogel 2021).

MILLENNIALS

Millennials are known by several different names including Gen Y, Next Generation, Net Generation, and Generation Me (Evans and Forbes 2012; Seemiller and Grace 2019b; Srinivasan 2012). While Seemiller and Grace (2019b) pose that Millennials were born from 1981 through 1994, other scholars pose their birth years between 1982 and 2002 (Coomes and DeBard

2004; Howe and Strauss 2003; Miller and Mills 2019). However, while there may be some disagreement regarding the length of generations, researchers identify similar characteristics and traits among the cohort. Millennials were raised during a time of globalization and evolving technology, further shaped by natural disasters and terrorist attacks. It is not surprising that they view themselves as globally educated, displaying assertive personality traits that portray confident individuals who expect to be successful (Chen and Choi 2008; Seemiller and Grace 2019b; Srinivasan 2012). This global awareness has also created a generation focused on the various dangers and threats that can occur, thus resulting in increased awareness and appreciation regarding the role of law enforcement.

When considering the generation that preceded them, Millennials represent a sharp break from Generation X (Gen Xers). However, this significant deviation is not uncommon. While Millennials rejected the behaviors and traits of Gen Xers (1961–1981), they did identify with the G.I. Generation (1901–1924). Early scholars found that when asked they spoke highly of this generation, often stating that they accomplished great things and helped to build a stronger nation (Howe and Strauss 2003).

As with every generation, Millennials have core traits that serve as the persona of the generation. These seven core traits include achieving, confident, conventional, pressured, sheltered, special, and team-oriented (Howe and Strauss 2000; Howe and Strauss 2003). Yet, while these traits are often how scholars describe this generation, not every generation member will exhibit them. Generational research should provide educators with information about their learners but should not dictate behavior. The goals of this research are to help educators gain a better perspective of, provide insights into, and provide a better understanding of their learners' preferences.

Personal Identity and Family Life

Millennials were one of the most diverse generations in history with early data showing that one in five Millennials had at least one parent who was an immigrant (Howe and Strauss 2003). This diversity resulted in a cohort that viewed themselves as being more global than their predecessors, embracing the diversity of their generation, and setting a tone of inclusivity with a focus on teams. They are often referred to as the "sunshine" generation as a result of having an easier childhood than their parents (Howe and Strauss 2003).

"Millennial children were the focal point of the family dynamic" (Gerhardt, Nachemson-Ekwall, and Fogel 2021, 36). While Gen Xers were latch-key kids, Millennials were doted upon, with their patents adjusting their schedules around childhood activities. Furthermore, Millennials actively sought love from their parents, and felt that their parents were easy to talk to (Howe and

Strauss 2003). This increased parental involvement impacted Millennials' development of independent decision making. They were less likely to go out on their own, drive a car, or hold a job. Because they looked to their parents as co-decision makers or to make the decision for them, Millennials struggle as their transition into college or as they enter the job market. As they had not dealt with life issues up to this point, educators and human resource managers are now expected to talk with parents rather than the student or employee. Furthermore, while Millennials are one of the most educated generations in history, their lack of self-direction has left them requiring significant guidance (Gerhardt, Nachemson-Ekwall, and Fogel 2021).

Personal expression is an important characteristic of this generation. Tattoos and piercings are prominent with 38% of Millennials having at least one tattoo and 23% having piercings in places other than their ears (Pew Research 2014; Shatto and Erwin 2017). This need for self-expression can result in issues when engaging with others from differing generations as those from other generations may view this self-expression with lacking professionalism.

Rule Followers and Expectations in Higher Education

Unlike the Gen Xers and Boomers before, Millennials embraced the idea of rules and regulations. Rather than push back against the institution, Millennials look to their parents, government, and institutions to set the expectations. Howe and Strauss note that Millennials embrace the idea of "social rules and standards" as it equates to an easier life (2003, 52). Moreover, they trust that large organizations will do the right thing while also recognizing that their own choices and actions are also important. The idea of individualism is the idea of authority (Howe and Strauss 2003). They tend to expect harsh punishments for those violating policies and laws.

This expectation of an organized approach to life extends to social events, activities, and learning. Millennials experienced an assessment-driven learning environment. This rigorous assessment approach to learning has extended into higher education, with many expecting faculty to integrate rubrics and specific learning goals into their courses. Furthermore, this educational foundation has resulted in Millennials entering higher education with their own clearly delineated learning goals and expected outcomes they presume to obtain prior to graduating (Miller and Mills 2019). Millennials are considered to be one of the most educated generations to date; Seemiller and Grace (2019b) found that 40% of those aged 20 to 29 years earned a bachelor's degree.

However, this assessment-driven education has provided Millennials with limited opportunities to fail academically prior to entering higher education.

As such, educators should be mindful that this generation may not be as resilient when academically challenged or when given limited feedback on a less successful academic endeavor. This generation expects clear and precise feedback, an understanding of the applicability of what they are learning to the career they have chosen, and a faculty member who is engaged within the learning environment (Miller and Mills 2019). Gone are the days where a "sage on the stage" was an acceptable approach to teaching. Chapter 5 will expand upon the role of the learning environment in more detail.

Leadership and Activism

Yet, while Millennials are typically rule followers, they do not look at their leaders with such blind devotion. "Millennials straddle the line between respecting authority and feeling that leadership is out of touch" (Phillips 2019, 15). They gravitate to leaders who strive to include them in the decision-making process and respond negatively to those leaders who exert power over others solely dependent on their positions. Leaders who promise the world and fail to deliver will lose the trust of this generation. Creating an environment that welcomes their contributions will foster productivity; if they are ignored their productivity will dwindle and will continue to decrease over time with every instance that they felt slighted or ignored (Phillips 2019).

Their activism extends to the environment and mental health issues. Most Millennials feel tied to the environment, focusing on "sustaining and preserving resources" as well as placing "emphasis on reducing consumption and recycling raw materials, and prioritize maintaining an environmentally friendly balance of using natural resources" (Phillips 2019, 89). This generation is also cognizant of the importance of maintaining good emotional and mental health. Advocating for access to counseling services has been a consistent goal of this generation as they navigate their collegiate experiences (Howe and Strauss 2003).

Relationships

Millennials also expect to engage with their peers and receive feedback from them as well. Peer relationships are important to Millennials and the idea of positive peer pressure is common within this generation. Peers expect their leaders to exhibit maturity and friendliness, while displaying a character of quality. While peer pressure is still present, it is not always seen as negative as scholars have found that it has pushed students to be more competitive, thus encouraging them to be their best selves through résumé building (Howe and Strauss 2003).

Millennials value friendships above most things, socializing in groups and using technology to remain connected. The growing popularity of texting and gaming during this generation's developmen, allows them to remain connected and to interact with multiple individuals at once, instead of one at a time. The relationship between Millennials and their parents is one of mutual understanding. They share similar tastes as their parents and find them easy to talk with regarding their hopes and concerns. This close relationship has led to parents being overly involved, often referred to as helicopter parents (Howe and Strauss 2003; Miller and Mills 2019; Seemiller and Grace 2019a) or lawnmower parents known for eliminating any problem that their children encounter. This closeness has led to separation anxiety, pushing institutions to identify ways to include parents as their children navigate their college journey. A more in-depth look at how institutions of higher education support learners will be featured in later chapters.

This close parental relationship has proven essential as Millennials have attained substantial student loan debt, resulting in their reliance on their parents well into early adulthood (Seemiller and Grace 2019b). This debt has also led many Millennials to delay marriage, children, and home ownership. Instead, they strive to identify mechanisms to economize, choosing to elect for ride shares instead of car ownership and reducing self-ownership of homes. They also tend to limit their purchases of material items, electing to use their funds to purchase experiences.

Role Models and Mentoring

"Mentor in Greek means to 'advise wisely' and is one who shows intent, purpose, spirit, and passion when helping others" (Evans and Forbes 2012, 397). Role modeling and mentorship is crucial when engaging with Millennial learners. They look for a mentoring relationship that is active and engaging and occurs consistently. Furthermore, they do not feel that a mentoring dynamic is limited to the traditional mentoring relationship. Instead, they look for those mentors or role models that are going to evaluate their needs and create a mentorship experience unique to them (Evans and Forbes 2012). To achieve this goal, Millennials want to have open dialogues regarding career opportunities and the tools they will need to support the professional growth needed to achieve these goals. Yet, they do not expect these dialogues to be one-directional. They look for mentors who are willing to create a partnership so that the overall mentoring experience is a positive one.

Health and Well-Being

As Millennials began entering college, teen behaviors of drinking, smoking, and drug use were on the decline. Howe and Strauss (2003) associated this change with the zero-tolerance expectations that began during their high school years and allowed many institutions of higher education to implement smoke-free campuses during this period with limited pushback from the student population.

Exposed to the importance of seeking help during their formative years, Millennials were more prone to seek medical solutions for ailments than previous generations (Howe and Strauss 2003). As such, Millennials viewed access to health services as an essential expectation within the college or university environment. The increasing number of students with diagnoses of attention deficit disorder (ADD), attention deficit hyperactivity disorder (ADHD), and asthma saw an increasing need for direct access to health services on campus; this trend pushed institutions to broaden student services to allow students to seek prescription renewals and medical attention without leaving campus.

Along with access to medical care, institutions also saw an increasing need for counseling services. Throughout Millennials' formative years there had been increased attention dedicated to emotional and psychiatric issues. While these mental health issues were less predominant in the older cohort of this generation, there were an increasing number of students seeking those services at both the high school and college levels, thus resulting in students regularly taking medications that required prescriptions and monitoring (Howe and Strauss 2003). This trend required colleges and universities to reevaluate the student services offered. This positive approach to mental health allowed groups of students who may not have been successful in previous generations to navigate the college experience successfully.

Preferences in the Workplace

Preparing learners to enter the workforce can be challenging, especially when considering the diverse makeup of generational cohorts currently working. This dynamic is even more complex when considering those working within the health professions. The following sections will provide a brief overview of preferences, with a deeper examination occurring in Chapter 10.

As of 2016, Millennials became the largest generation in the workforce in the United States (Fry 2018). As they entered the workforce, many had not previously held jobs. As teens, the number of Millennials working greatly decreased. This lack of work experience prior to college may have resulted from parental and teacher influence. As this generation was navigating their formative years, one-third of teens reported receiving funds for extraneous purchases from parents and/or grandparents. This generation is known for establishing the "nag factor," which resulted in teens requesting money multiple times until funds were secured to purchase items (Howe and Strauss 2003).

This culture change was also the result of changes in parental expectations. Rather than have their children work, parents (and teachers) pushed them to focus on getting into a good college. This required Millennials to focus more on community service, athletics, and experiences that built a résumé. This lack of interest in employment could have also resulted from minimized time available; this generation saw significant increases in time needed for school, after-school programming, chores, personal care, and travel (Howe and Strauss 2003). Lastly, for those that did seek employment, Millennials gravitated to positions that allowed for skills training or specialization.

When Millennials enter the job market, they tend to gravitate to positions that provide autonomy and freedom (Shatto and Erwin 2016). They also look for job opportunities that they see as interesting and meaningful. Phillips (2019) found that there are three drivers that create engagement with Millennials: (1) serving a valuable purpose; (2) being empowered to deliver results; and (3) working in a fulfilling environment. These drivers provide the leverage needed to support Millennials to be the best versions of themselves in the work environment. Millennials want to see how their actions impact the greater good and move beyond their own personal benefit. Having the ability to see how their contributions align with the success of the organization spurs them on to continue working and striving for success. Furthermore, they want to work in environments that create positive energy, fosters inspiration, hosts a strong culture, and allows for work-balance. If these characteristics are present, money is less of a driving force (Phillips 2019).

However, should a Millennial fail to see those opportunities in their current place of employment, they will not limit themselves to simply changing jobs if they feel unfulfilled; instead, they will change careers if they feel it will result in a more fulfilling existence (Taylor 2018). To achieve this fulfillment, Millennials will look to workplace role models for coaching and mentoring, expecting a personal relationship (Taylor 2018; Delgado et al. 2020). "Millennials often entered the work world expecting that their voices would matter to the same extent for their bosses" (Gerhardt, Nachemson-Ekwall, and Fogel 2021, 37). Yet, while they rely on their parents for their own personal guidance, Millennials often feel confident to take on higher levels of responsibilities with less experience. This has created friction in the work pace, as many of those from earlier generations do not feel that Millennials understand that they need to wait their turn to succeed. Millennials will also expect work–life balance and will value this over prestige and money

(Delgado et al. 2020). This need for work–life balance does not equate to being averse to hard work.

CHAPTER SUMMARY AND CONCLUSION

Generational theory provides educators with a better understanding of students in today's classroom. While each generation may have its own unique characteristics, how these characteristics are shaped is cyclical in nature. Most generations are influenced by worldwide events such as war, terrorism, economic challenges, and so forth. As such, there is value in looking to the past to see how future generations will be shaped.

Millennials' transition into college resulted in the revitalization of higher education and created a plethora of data examining how educators could best support their learning journeys. These studies demonstrated the importance of understanding the needs and expectations of each new generation of learners and prompted educators to reexamine how they engage with each new generational cohort. Chapter 2 examines Generation Z and the expectations this generation has as they navigate higher education and transition into the workforce. Last, it explores how Millennials and Gen Zs are similar and different, and how educators should navigate multigenerational learners within the educational setting.

Chapter 2

Generation Z Enters Higher Education and How They Compare to Millennials

The transition from Millennials to Generation Z in undergraduate education has been well established; however, Millennials continue to reengage within higher education at the graduate and doctoral levels. "The generational diversity in higher education presents unique challenges to engagement and retention of students, as many of the common attitudes and tendencies of the undergraduates are not congruent with those expected by the faculty teaching their courses" (Miller and Mills 2019, 79). While this quote by Miller and Mills speaks to the generational differences between students and faculty, the same is true for those multigenerational students in the classroom or clinical experience. Navigating the multigenerational terrain can be challenging for all those involved, so it is critical that educators be aware of how to best support this diverse group of learners. This chapter will examine how Gen Zs navigate the world around them as well as explore how this generation's expectations align and differ from Millennials.

GENERATION Z

Opinions vary regarding the initial birth years for Generation Z (Gen Z). Seemiller and Grace (2019a) pose that Gen Zs were born in 1995 through 2010, clearly aligning the 9/11 terrorist attack with the oldest Gen Zs. Chicca and Shellenbarger (2018) consider Gen Z birth years as mid-1990s to 2012, while Pew Research Center (2019) notes 1997 as the first year of this generations birth, with others indicating that Gen Zs were born in the early 2000s (Miller and Mills 2019; Shatto and Erwin 2016). As discussed in Chapter 1, many feel that labeling a generation by birth years is limiting and should be defined by the shared economic, social, and cultural factors that shaped the generation (Wilkins 2021). Seemiller and Grace (2019a) note that "[i]n many cases, though, the start and/or end dates put forth by different entities are usually only off from each other 1 to 2 years, leaving the remaining years in the middle the same" (xviii–xix). The overlapping nature of generational traits also impacts scholars' abilities to clearly delineate birth years.

When examining how Generation Z learners engage within higher education, it is important to recognize that existing research focuses primarily on the elder cohort of this generation. For example, Seemiller and Grace (2019a) delineate Gen Zs into two groups, Big Z (born 1995 to 2002) and Little Z (born 2003 to 2010). For their research, they tend to focus on those born between 1995 and 2002 as this subgroup represents the older generation and more existing data are available. As time progresses, academic researchers may begin to see different characteristics and traits emerge as Generation Alpha (the next generation) enters their teenage years.

Personal Identity and Family Life

Gen Zs are even more uniquely diverse than Millennials (Wilkins 2021), with researchers noting that they are increasing biracial or multiracial (Miller and Mills 2019; Seemiller and Grace 2016; Shatto and Erwin 2016;). Forty-nine percent of Gen Zs identify as non-white (Seemiller and Grace, 2019a). However, their race and ethnicity are not the only characteristics that make them unique; the diversity of family make-ups is also growing, with many Gen Zs having same-sex parents as well as parents from diverse backgrounds and cultures (Shatto and Erwin 2016). Gen Zs also report high rates of non-heterosexual orientation and acceptance of gender fluid identification. A study found that only 48% of Gen Zs identified as heterosexual and 81% indicated that their gender did not identify them (Seemiller and Grace, 2019a).

The personal diversity of these individuals has made this generation more open and inclusive than previous generations, to include Millennials (Shatto and Erwin 2016; Wilkins 2021). They welcome diversity and embrace the growing diversity within the United States (Seemiller and Grace 2016) and strive to be open minded and inclusive to create an environment of equality (Seemiller and Grace 2019a). "Generation Z's open views on gender will likely propel them front and center in discussions around policies and practices related to gender identity, especially as they move into decision-making roles in adulthood" (Seemiller and Grace 2016, 113).

Social media also serves as an extension of themselves, portraying one identity online while displaying an entirely different persona in real life. Gen Zs are comfortable managing multiple online identities at once and can cultivate their identities utilizing the settings available in each type of social media platform to create the identity they want others to see. Snapchat has been their go-to social media platform as it served as one of the first platforms created that was not carried over from previous generations. Gen Zs also embrace Instagram as the privacy settings allow them to cultivate their personas, protecting their real identity from others. This generation often hosts two accounts, their "Rinsta" (public account with a cultivated identity and lots of followers) and their "Finsta" (private account shared with friends) to allow them to present two different versions of themselves to the world (Seemiller and Grace 2019a).

However, the duality of these identities also impacts how they see themselves. Many Gen Zs rate their self-confidence lower than their intellect (Seemiller and Grace 2019a). While digital technology allows Gen Zs to make friends all over the world, many still identify as feeling lonely. Seemiller and Grace (2019a) found that a significant number of Gen Zs report feeling shy, isolated, alone, unknown, and unseen even when surrounded by others. While the social community they build online gives the impression of being supported by friends and likeminded peers, these online friendships cannot substitute for the benefits of face-to-face engagement.

Impact of Technology and the Internet

As we began to see with Millennials, Gen Zs have lived their lives with extreme exposure to media, especially social media. The internet has always been readily available for this generation and has allowed Gen Zs to be inundated with constant video uploads, tweets, and posts since their birth. Every minute, 2.5 million new posts/articles/uploads appear on Facebook®, along with 100,000 tweets on X (formally known as Twitter), and 49 hours of new content appearing on YouTube (Daugherty and Hoffman 2014; Shatto and Erwin 2016). Gen Zs have always had access to social media, which has further solidified their feelings of global-connectedness and a constant feeling of connectedness with people. Further, this access to instant information has impacted the way this generation navigates the everyday world as they have never had to wait for information to become available. This generation is the first to be raised with smartphones, which has prepared them to do everything on one device; whereas previous generations had to navigate multiple devices at a time (Seemiller and Grace 2016). On average, Gen Zs spend nine hours a day on their cellphones (Shatto and Erwin 2016). Gen Zs are the first generation to grow up with services such as YouTube and Netflix, which allows for on-demand streaming, thus allowing this generation to filter and absorb information on their own timetables (Shatto and Erwin 2016).

While social media and the internet have greatly influenced this generation, they are not the only influencers. This generation has also been shaped by the advent of handheld devices and smartphones. Access is no longer limited to a desktop computer or even a laptop. Rather, Gen Zs have instant access to the internet and all their social media accounts all day, every day through their tablets or smartphones. Yet, while these devices can serve as positive influences (i.e., access to much needed resources such as law enforcement and mental health services), they have also allowed for increased mechanisms for bullying, specifically cyber bullying. Screen time has also impacted social and oral communication skills. While Gen Zs prefer a virtual environment, it has been shown to increase feelings of isolation and insecurity, perpetuating the likelihood for mental health issues (Chicca and Shellenbarger 2018; Wilkins 2021).

This access to information and technology impacts the way this generation learns and thus affects the way educators must approach teaching. Gen Z brains have been programmed to understand complex visual images, which supports their need for visual teaching approaches and why those teaching strategies are more effective (Hallowell and Ratey 2011; Shatto and Erwin 2016). Considered to be self-directed learners, integrating technology should help Gen Zs thrive in the learning environment. Access to constant information has shaped how they approach learning, with Gen Zs using things such as YouTube to observe a skill prior to practicing it. This trend of observation and practice has carried forward into the learning environment with many Gen Zs preferring this method to the previously established reading and listening approach, which has been commonplace in higher education. This need for instant gratification creates a level of frustration in this generation when answers are not readily available or the content being relayed is unclear (Shatto and Erwin 2016).

Unfortunately, this instant access has resulted in decreased attention span moving from 12 seconds for Millennials to 8 seconds for Gen Zs with some scholars associating this decline as acquired attention deficit disorder (Miller and Mills 2019; Shatto and Erwin 2016). However, while their attention spans may be dwindling, their ability to navigate technology has increased. As such, educators should consider having students create videos related to the course content and adding opportunities for peer feedback to increase critical thinking skills for both the creator and reviewer.

Relationships

Studies have found that Gen Zs see themselves as loyal, thoughtful, determined, compassionate, open minded, and responsible (Seemiller and Grace 2016; Seemiller and Grace 2019a). Dr. Candace Steele Flippin's work *Generation Z in the Workplace* found that they describe themselves as eager, hardworking, creative, and motivated (2017). A study conducted by the VIA

Institute on Character found Gen Z strengths to include honesty, kindness, humor, fairness, and judgment (VIA Institute on Character 2018). However, when asked to describe their peers, Gen Zs tend to view them more harshly than themselves, describing their peers as competitive, spontaneous, adventuresome, and curious (Seemiller and Grace 2016; Seemiller and Grace 2019a). The relationship Gen Zs have with their peers is dynamic, with peers serving as one of their main influencers providing the advice and support needed to navigate the world around them (Seemiller and Grace 2019). Peer influencers are not just those physically near them but can also be present in online communities and social groups. Often, Gen Zs will identify with peers that host video blogs or Instagram accounts looking to these peers for advice about products or services.

While they look to their peers for guidance, Gen Z learners favor intrapersonal learning (Seemiller and Grace 2016). As they prefer to be self-reliant when learning, if tasked with working with a group or team, they would rather select their team and divide the work among team members so it can be completed independently. This trait is one shared with Millennials; however, how they approach the team meeting differs. Millennials tended to avoid meeting in person, Gen Z learners are open to meeting if needed, using this time to work independently on their sections while sitting silently side-by-side using a Google Doc or some other type of electronic information gathering document (Seemiller and Grace 2016).

Role Models and Mentoring

Gen Zs place an increased importance on role models and mentoring. Prior to college, many Gen Zs have focused their attentions on personal achievements, primarily within academics, focusing less on extracurricular activities, which were of great importance to Millennials. They have focused primarily on personal and professional skill development, achieved through focused internships or volunteer opportunities, and strategic thinking. Each personal choice was made after considering how each choice could impact their future trajectory. This focus has created a generation striving to do well in life but who have limited experience being unsuccessful or failing to meet their goals. Furthermore, this laser focus has created a populous that fears failure and lacks confidence when navigating new challenges (Wilkins 2021). This lack of experience will push Gen Zs to seek out mentors/role models who can prepare them for the journey ahead and provide them with the skills needed to successfully navigate their careers. Yet, while Gen Zs are adept at considering the ramifications of personal choices, the influence and increased utilization of social media has created challenges within this generation's ability to determine professional and appropriate practices, with many grappling to understand how their digital lives can impact their future careers (Wilkins 2021). As such, role models and mentors should be prepared to navigate these challenging dialogues, lending guidance as to how one's online persona impacts their professional one.

Seemiller and Grace (2019a) note that Gen Zs place increased value on relationships, especially relationships with mentors. As career-minded individuals, they tend to gravitate toward educational experiences that will support them in their future professions (Hampton and Keys 2016; Seemiller and Grace 2019a; Wilkins 2021). Yet, as this generation has typically entered college without holding a job, they may enter the workforce lacking any work experience and may require more direct guidance and mentoring as a result (Chicca and Shellenbarger 2018; Schenarts 2020; Schroth 2019; Wilkins 2021). They "desire seasoned mentors whom they respect and will be eager to learn from a caring faculty member or practitioner" (Wilkins 2021, 31). The positive parental relationships Gen Zs have experienced has created a generation expecting supportive relationships within the professional work environment. As such, they are open to engaging with mentors that genuinely care about their success and want to support them as they navigate the professional world.

As such, the importance placed on mentoring and role modeling relationships correlates with this generation's preference for experiential learning. As Gen Zs expect to learn practical skills required for their future careers, experiential learning allows the learner to work closely with a practitioner in the field, receiving timely and targeted feedback. Their appreciation for hands-on learning allows them to successfully connect with their mentors, thus further building the relationship (Wilkins 2021). Furthermore, they will strive to prove themselves to their mentors as they fear disappointing them (Seemiller and Grace 2016). Yet, while positive role models and mentoring relationships are important to this generation, Gen Zs lack respect for those mentors or role models that do not seek out or consider how they can contribute to the relationship as well as the learning or working environment (Seemiller and Grace 2016).

Activism and Leadership

Gen Zs, to a greater degree than Millennials, value advocacy and activism (Seemiller and Grace 2019a). They are oriented toward social change and much more likely to volunteer their time to make a difference. However, they have a general dislike of formal positional leadership. They have a general belief that politicians are dishonest, selfish, and argumentative, and as a result these feelings often impact their willingness to hold positions within student organizations (Seemiller and Grace 2017b). Yet, while they host these negative feelings toward political leadership, Gen Zs expect the government to play a prominent role in solving societal problems (Parker and Igielnik 2020) like racism and economy-related issues.

College for many Gen Zs is a mechanism to cultivate leaders and promote awareness of social issues. Colleges also offer a front row seat to marches, rallies, boycotts, and demonstrations, as well as a collection of others willing to participate in these activities (Seemiller and Grace 2019a). The Class of 2022 fall survey conducted by Niche found that 63% of students said that personalized and meaningful communal outreach made an influential impact in their consideration to apply or attend that institution (Patch 2021).

While Gen Zs are committed to advocating for change, this generation has an over inflated sense of their own leadership skills, often thinking poorly of others regarding their leadership abilities while feeling that their own leadership skills are more than competent. Educators must be prepared to help foster the development of these skills to support this generations' development. To effectively achieve this charge, institutions will need to carefully consider how they engage Gen Zs in leadership opportunities, and it may require that institutions adopt a non-positional leadership model (Seemiller and Grace 2017b).

Seemiller and Grace (2017b) discuss the need to demonstrate to Gen Zs the value associated with participating in leadership opportunities as these students are not interested in joining or leading organizations simply for the opportunity to make friends, as previous generations had been willing to do in the past. Seemiller and Grace (2017b) propose four critical value propositions that must be met to entice Gen Zs. These values include the development of ethical, positive, and caring leaders; the development of critical career competencies; the opportunity to pursue their passions; and finally, to make a difference (Seemiller and Grace 2017b). The integration of these four core values will speak to this generation as it aligns with their need to leave the world in a better place than when they came into it.

When considering health professions students, the development of advocacy and leadership skills is crucial to support patient-centered care and quality outcomes. For example, the Hippocratic oath, an oath that medical students take upon graduation from medical school, is centered on the need to care for others from a humanistic standpoint. Caring for patients holistically and social activism go hand in hand. Paul relays this sentiment succinctly, stating, "In the current climate, the practice of healing is inextricably tied to the social and political context, such that advocacy and activism have become essential to a career in medicine" (Paul 2019, 1071). Those in Generation Z desire to make an impact, and thus rely on those in leadership to effect change. They want their college and career experiences to challenge the status quo (Seemiller and Grace 2019a). Within health professions programs, curricula that invests in the student experience will meet the needs of Generation Z. As such, clinical experiences that promote experiential learning, student life, and collaboration with other healthcare providers are desired by this generation of students. These aspects are explored in more depth in subsequent chapters in this text.

Overcoming a Cautious Nature

Gen Zs are often considered overly cautious in nature, tending to avoid challenges in which they may struggle or fail to succeed (Chicca and Shellenbarger 2018; Schenarts 2020; Wilkins 2021). While they value achievement and long-term goals, Gen Zs are often overly concerned with being successful, taking fewer potential risks and typically only with a back-up plan in place (Wilkins 2021). This generation has been encouraged to attain personal achievements, thus resulting in a generation that wants to do well in life but fears failure and lacks confidence.

Like Millennials before them, Gen Zs have been over parented, which has resulted in a slower transition into adulthood. Coomes and DeBard (2004) note that the youth stage within Strauss and Howe's model is one of dependence to include embracing the protection and safety afforded by one's parents. This hesitancy for Gen Zs to move into adulthood may be the result of improved relationships between parents and their Gen Z offspring. Many Gen Zs are delaying those first steps associated with independence such as learning to drive and seeking their first employment experiences; instead, they have continued to look to their parents to guide them through the decision-making process much longer than any previous generation. When considering Strauss and Howes's interpretation of generational progression, this developmental delay may influence how the next generation navigates the transition from youth to adulthood but at this time, it is too early to determine whether it will push Generation Alpha to seek independence or strive to remain in the youth stage longer.

Millennials were willing to embrace costs associated with college tuition as they aligned this achievement with future professional success and increased net worth. As a cohort, Gen Zs are more fiscally conservative than Millennials and when faced with the drastically increased costs for college tuition, many are evaluating the benefits of attending to the financial challenges that will be incurred. Between 2003 and 2013, college tuition increased 80% and Gen Zs are hyperaware of the significant debt Millennials have undertaken as a result. Furthermore, research has found that student loan debt and student success are correlated with increased student loan debt resulting in increased likelihood of student withdrawal (Seemiller and Grace 2019a). With these findings it is not surprising that Gen Zs tend to gravitate to institutions of higher education that allow flexibility in additional costs, preferring services to be offered a la cart so costs can be minimized. These trends as well as ongoing media coverage regarding the cost of college attendance has pushed Gen Zs to evaluate the rate of return on this fiscal investment (Seemiller and Grace 2019a). While the number of Gen Zs attending college is not the record numbers of the Millennial generation, many Gen Zs identify attending college as overly expensive but necessary. A more in-depth look at the financial ramifications of higher education will be explored in Chapter 3 of this book.

Communicating with Others

Gen Z's adoption of digital communication has eliminated the boundaries traditional communication methods have imposed; etiquette no longer dictates that communicating late at night is inappropriate (Seemiller and Grace 2019a). Furthermore, digital messaging has changed communication, removing an end point from the dialogue, and increasing the flexibility of communicating across platforms. However, this change has the potential to increase anxiety as users are then required to check all forms of social media, email, and text to ensure that they do not miss any portion of the discussion.

The communication methods Gen Zs use differs; however, they tend to gravitate toward face-to-face communication when possible and will utilize video chatting as an alternative when face-to-face is not an option (Seemiller and Grace 2017b). They prefer this communication method as it allows them to see non-verbal behaviors and facial expressions, thus providing insight into what the other individual is thinking and feeling. Gen Z's preference for face-to-face and in-person discussions may also be driven by their relationship goals. This generation seeks to have more than superficial connections as they look to their peers/friends to influence their life choices.

This generation gravitates toward texting as their preferred medium for communicating when face-to-face is not possible. They favor texting as it allows people to respond at their leisure, can be accomplished on the go, and the conversation can span longer periods of time or be ongoing. As smartphone users, Gen Zs use their devices on average 3 hours a day for texting (Seemiller and Grace 2019a).

This adoption of social/digital media has required the integration of new ways for expressing emotions, thus the advent of emoticons and eventually emojis. Gen Zs utilize emojis and GIFs to display emotions, with memes serving to connect to a topic or cultural reference. Yet, Gen Zs have taken memes one step further, creating their own individualized memes to express their individuality.

This generation is no longer limited by location when communicating with others and there are generational differences regarding when it is acceptable to use one's phone. Before Gen Zs, many would have balked at the idea of answering a call or text at important family events, church gatherings, or solemn occasions (Seemiller and Grace 2019a). Gen Zs interconnectedness with their peers changes their views of these communications, viewing them as mechanisms of support that should be acknowledged whenever they deem acceptable. Yet, how one communicates is not the only change that has occurred within this generation. What they deem as acceptable to discuss with others has also evolved. The days of oversharing on social media are gone as Gen Zs embrace the ramifications of widespread use of social media and the platform it creates. They are aware that a wider audience now has access to information that they share and can provide opportunities for them to vocalize opinions that previous generations may have been leery to discuss. While they accept social media as a platform to spread information to likeminded individuals, they also respect the negative ramifications social media can create if their opinions are misrepresented or taken out of context.

Health and Well-Being

"Generation Z students have had exposure to many large-scale high stress events during their lifetimes that have had the potential to contribute to personal fear and anxiety and the construction of unhealthy beliefs about themselves" (Seemiller and Grace 2016, 196). As a result, there is an increasing number of students entering into college with mental health issues. These Gen Z students may not seek out counseling because of the costs associated, limited availability of counselors, or the stigma attached to seeking assistance. To counteract this tendency, colleges and universities should consider offering counseling services at no cost to help support students. It will also be important for faculty and staff to engage students in regular discussions regarding the value of counseling to help off-set Gen Zs feelings that they will be stigmatized if they seek out those services.

Gen Zs have spent significant time online or on their devices, which has fostered feelings of isolation, insecurity, and increases the likelihood for mental health issues within this generation (Chicca and Shellenbarger 2018; Wilkins 2021). This increased screen time has impacted social and oral communication skills and have also resulted in a generation of sedentary individuals (Seemiller and Grace 2016). This generation was raised in a time where physical activity was on the decline with less outdoor activities during peak periods of growth. This lack of activity and tendency toward indoor activities has the potential to further exacerbate mental health issues as it will also impact feelings of isolation. Colleges and universities should be mindful of these tendencies and identify strategies for engaging students in real time outside of the virtual environment.

This generation has also shown concerns regarding their diet. They tend to gravitate to food choices that allow them to select organic choices or that align with a fresh diet (Seemiller and Grace 2016). Gen Zs also want their food to be produced in healthy, sustainable, and ethical manners. They were raised during a time when vegan, vegetarian, gluten-free, or lactose-free food options were readily available. Institutions should be mindful of dining choices available and ensure that there are plenty of healthy options to include food cooked to order as well as meals that include fresh fruits and vegetables.

Expectations in Higher Education

Gen Z students want a personalized college experience that will support them emotionally, mentally, and academically (Seemiller and Grace 2016). More than half of Gen Zs reported that the availability and convenience of campus facilities were an important factor in deciding where to attend college. Seeing college attendance as a joint responsibility between self and institution, more than 70% of Gen Zs desire to influence their chosen course of study to meet personal needs (Seemiller and Grace 2016). Campus support structures do not always meet the needs of Gen Z students. Often, student affairs and counseling services are delivered solely through a central office on campus, and therefore might not include the personal counseling, career counseling, mentorship opportunities, and inclusive and affirming environment that is necessitated by Gen Z students. Additionally, academic programs tend to favor on-campus experiences that minimize the potential of online or asynchronous learning opportunities valued by this generation.

Developing the whole student requires institutions to embrace innovative solutions. This is especially difficult within health professions, as the focus tends to be on training for patient care and less about the student experience. In a qualitative study conducted in a medical school, the breadth of the curriculum and non-interactive teaching approaches were contributing factors to maladjustment issues of medical students (Vimal et al. 2021). In response, the authors suggested stronger student support systems that emphasize the various roles of stakeholders. These initiatives include course orientations, mentorship programs, enhancing student wellness, counseling, conflict resolution, stronger study habits, and student-friendly environments.

A promising approach to improving the student experience, and ultimately student-centered outcomes, includes helping students comprehensively address the many personal and institutional barriers they face while in college. According to Dawson, Kearney, and Sullivan (2021a), there are four categories attributed to the non-completion rates among college students: (1) academic under-preparation, (2) high college tuition costs,

(3) institutional obstacles, and (4) personal non-academic obstacles (e.g., financial stresses, child-care, and transportation). These barriers are common among all college students, but they are especially perplexing for low-income students, as these are often the students with the most limited access to resources (Dawson, Kearney, and Sullivan, 2021a). As a result, more comprehensive support for all students' attending college is needed.

Generation Z in the Workplace

Within the work environment, Gen Zs will flourish in a structured and hierarchical environment that allows for fluidity and flexibility. This flexibility and fluidity pertain primarily to their active participation and engagement across all levels of the organization (Seemiller and Grace 2016). Furthermore, while Gen Zs expect their leaders to listen to what they have to say, they recognize that their leaders will have final say over important matters.

Like the Millennials before them, many Gen Zs may enter the workforce with limited experience and require more direct guidance and mentoring. Those that elect to enter traditional careers will look for employment that they view as meaningful and which will allow them to make a difference (Wilkins 2021). Gen Zs reliance on technology and their need to remain connected will serve them well as they enter the professional world. They will look for employment opportunities that allow the flexibility they desire, which includes alternate scheduling, project-based opportunities, and self-defined work hours. They will also look for versatility regarding where they can work; this generation prefers to not only set their own hours but to work from wherever they happen to be at the time. Only 28% of Gen Zs prefer to work in a traditional office space as compared to 46% of Millennials (Seemiller and Grace 2016).

The increasing number of self-employment opportunities available during Gen Zs development has also influenced how they view their future careers. They have been raised during a time where self-employment and creative entrepreneurship allowed individuals to "rent, sell, or serve others without owning a business," which allowed them to establish their own terms and conditions for the products and services they offered (Seemiller and Grace 2016, 31). Job opportunities such as Uber, Taskrabbit, and now YouTube, have taught Gen Zs that a career no longer has limitations. They can create the jobs they want that allow them to have the lifestyle they prefer.

NAVIGATING GENERATIONAL SIMILARITIES AND DIFFERENCES

As with every generation, Millennials and Generation Z have varying outlooks on their personal and professional lives. Yet, there are also similarities between these generations that should not be ignored. Both Millennials and Gen Zs strive to have happy and successful lives. It is in their approach where they divide. Whether because of college debt incurred or preference, Millennials create a culture of sharing to include living spaces and car services. While not opposed to sharing services when they are convenient, Gen Zs strive to own their own homes and vehicles. Seemiller and Grace (2019a) associate this trend with this generation's need for freedom and convenience.

Both generations were considered more diverse than the ones before them. With Millennials, diversity regarding race and ethnicity were the primary focus. Gen Zs are not only more racially and ethnically diverse, but they are also living in homes with more diverse familial pairings, which include same-sex parents, multigenerational, or single-parent situations (Shatto and Erwin 2016). Gen Zs acceptance of those different from themselves further shapes this generation's uniqueness. Considered to be more open-minded than even Millennials, Gen Zs are more accepting of sexual orientation, gender fluidity, religious differences, and diverse viewpoints, and expect to have a diverse group of friends.

Adapting the Classroom for Learners of Multiple Generations

Over the next decade, it will be essential to create a learning environment that meets the needs of Millennial and Gen Z learners. With the dwindling number of students graduating from high school, higher education will need to attract Millennial learners back to colleges and universities to finish their undergraduate degrees, to supplement their degrees through graduate education, or to support professional development opportunities through certificate programs or microcredentials. However, to achieve this, faculty will need to identify and address the different expectations these learners will have within the learning environment (Miller and Mills 2019).

Neither Millennials nor Gen Z learners anticipate the challenges they will face during the transition into higher education; these challenges are often personal, social, as well as academic. Often both generations fail to realize that their college or university experience will differ from what they have previously experienced and that there is increased potential for them to be academically unsuccessful. Miller and Mills note that college/university is their first opportunity to "fail academically in a context with little direct parental involvement and more distant teachers than in high school" (2019, 80). As a result, these learners will look for institutions that have faculty who care about them as individuals but also about their ability to be successful.

A key consideration for higher education administrators as they strive to entice both generations into their institutions are the differing levels of expectations each generation possesses. Gen Z learners are more financially driven and practical than Millennials, with many expressing that a degree from a college or university is not necessary to navigate a successful career (Seemiller and Grace 2016). Higher education administrators should be prepared to see a decreasing number of Gen Z applicants as a result.

Role of Faculty and Mentoring

A key area to address for both Millennials and Gen Zs is the role of faculty within the learning environment. Scholars have found that the role of faculty caring and student learning in higher education is essential for student success and retention (Meyers 2011; Slate et al. 2011). Miller and Mills found that there was "a clear emphasis on faculty caring as an important factor for these Millennial and Generation Z students' motivation and engagement in learning" (2019, 78). They noted that instructors need to emphasize their ability to communicate empathically to increase student success and to create a culture of student learning and persistence. As a result, if they feel that their faculty care about them, students are more likely to strive to be academically successful. These generations need frequent interactions as well as guidance regarding both personal and academic challenges. Furthermore, they need to feel that their instructors are fair and encouraging while displaying a basic understanding of what is happening in their students' personal lives.

A key factor in student engagement and persistence is creating a sense of caring within higher education (Miller and Mills 2019). Studies have found that students who feel that their instructors care have shown increased motivation, are more likely to engage in the classroom, and find their instructors more credible (Chory and Offstein 2017; Finn et al. 2009; Miller and Mills 2019; Slate et al. 2011). Miller and Mills (2019) conducted a study at a regional institution to better understand what caring looks like for Millennial and Gen Z learners. They found alignment between caring as a personality and how an instructor approached teaching. While one's teaching technique does matter, students did not limit how they ascertained a faculty member's level of caring. They associated caring with both attitude and/or demeanor as well as pedagogical classroom practices. Respondents indicated that good teaching could override an instructor's bad attitude or demeanor, indicating that good teaching demonstrated a sense of caring even if the instructor's attitude did not.

These findings may challenge some faculty as many may view this as negating their roles as educators, which requires some distance between themselves and their students to be objective regarding academic progress. Others may view this expectation as an increased burden or a lack of student maturity, thus creating a level of faculty pushback due to increased workloads with limited or no additional compensation. Yet, faculty must recognize that the concept of caring has additional ramifications. Institutions with faculty and staff that fail to be seen as caring will struggle to retain students and will be challenged with identifying alternative strategies for supporting student success.

Teaching Multigenerational Learners

Identifying strategies for reaching multigenerational learners is increasingly complex due to the diversity of higher education; faculty consist of members of the following generations: "Silent" generation, Baby Boomers, Generation X, and Millennials (Miller and Mills 2019). The student population is comprised primarily of Millennial and Generation Z learners. This diversity creates challenges for faculty and staff as they must identify strategies for student engagement and retention that may not align with their preferences. Miller and Mills (2019) associate this disjointedness with some of the more negative generational traits, such as entitlement or unpreparedness, used to describe both generations.

Both Millennials and Gen Zs expect their faculty to create linkages between what they are learning and the real-world environment. They expect instructors to be relatable and create a genuine experience. These learning environments should engage students and include innovative teaching approaches such as narratives, storytelling, social media, and so forth (Shatto and Erwin 2017). The integration of relatable entities is also key with Miller and Mills (2019) suggesting the importance of integrating examples from pop culture to help instill meaning in the learning experience. Furthermore, both generations prefer to observe and practice skills (Chicca and Shellenbarger 2018; Shatto and Erwin 2016; Wilkins 2021); as such, faculty should be prepared to allow students the hands-on learning they crave to keep them engaged within the learning environment.

Additionally, both generations expect faculty to engage in adaptive teaching strategies to ensure that they recognize where students are academically. The inclusion of adaptive teaching approaches incorporates the integration of active learning strategies such as flipped classrooms, fieldwork experiences, and so forth. Millennials and Gen Zs expect rapidly changing technology and for technology to be integrated throughout the learning environment (Shatto and Erwin 2017). Lastly, this responsive approach to teaching should ensure that students have the opportunity to provide feedback to support educators as they adapt the learning environment to meet the learning needs of their students.

MILLENNIALS AND GENERATION Z WITHIN HEALTH PROFESSIONS EDUCATION

Millennials and Generation Z have similar and differing expectations within the learning environment that amplifies the need to identify strategies for educating both generational cohorts. When considering health professions education, this additional layer poses further challenges as educators are tasked with navigating a multigenerational learning environment to prepare the next generation of health practitioners with the knowledge and skills needed to navigate not only the traditional classroom but the complexities of the clinical environment. The following sections will provide a brief overview as to the dynamic landscape of health professions education within a multigenerational learning environment, but this topic will be explored in greater detail in later chapters.

Identifying key teaching approaches is just one element of the bigger puzzle. While creating an inclusive and dynamic learning environment is vital, learners must also be challenged outside the classroom as well. Both generations are aggrieved by assignments viewed as busy work or lacking any real value to future practice (Mohr and Mohr 2017). Clear alignment between assignments and/or experiences with future practice will be key to keeping learners engaged. The integration of technology into the learning environment has been well established for both generations and will be expected to allow learners access to the most up-to-date information available. Yet, the integration of technology into the learning environment should be intentional and include adequate student training. This additional training is essential to ensure that learners understand the role of confidentiality and privacy of patients, and also addresses the ramifications of patient disclosures across information sharing platforms (Shatto and Erwin 2017).

For Gen Z and Millennial students, their digital connectiveness plays a large part in their learning preferences and idiosyncrasies. They seek rapid gratification and have short attention spans. The average attention span of Gen Z students regarding classroom learning is estimated to be only 7 to 10 minutes (Szymkowiak et al. 2021). They seek immediacy in solving problems and answering questions. As a result, they value access to information over quality of information, and tend to multi-task due to the need for stimulation. This has important implications for students, as information found on the web may lack credibility.

Both Millennial and Gen Z students are career focused. As a result, the educational experience they receive in college matters to them. They value immersive experiences that equip them for a career. Millennials are a highly educated generation, frequently wanting things that are bigger and better (Seemiller and Grace 2016). High-paying careers, like medical-related fields, are often sought by Millennials and Gen Zs (Seemiller and Grace 2016; Seemiller and Grace 2019a). Pursuing a degree in a medical field is enticing because it offers job security with the ability to make a high income suitable for today's living standards.

A health professions career, which tends to be highly experiential and skills-focused, is a path that fulfills the tactile needs of these generations. This is especially true for Gen Z learners, who are more practical than Millennials. Gen Z's need for hands-on experiences could be due in part to their need for quick information processing (Zarra 2017).

Generational Theory and Generational Humility in Health Professions Education

Generational theory is well established within the health professions education literature; however, some question how this theoretical framework creates bias within educators. Jauregui et al. (2019) postulated the elimination of generational theory within health professions education and the integration of the concept of generational humility. The authors note that educators may use their observations and trainees to create generational assumptions, thus establishing their own bias regarding motives instead of looking at learner expectations based on their own merits or values. By adopting the idea of generational humility, Jauregui et al. propose that this "approach in which critical consciousness and humility are used to explore the unique needs, values, and motivations of learners" will allow educators to respond to the identified needs of the learner (2019, 63). While generational humility strives to replace generational theory as an appropriate framework, it is possible for the two frameworks to work in tandem to provide educators with a variety of resources which will allow them to support their learners.

Role of Professionalism and Professional Identity Formation

Millennials and Gen Zs have varying expectations as to how they intend to navigate their professional lives. These differences may prove challenging when navigating how to foster and promote professional identity formation and professionalism within these cohorts. The role of professionalism is an ongoing concern within health professions education, with many disciplines still navigating their definition of professionalism and how to successfully evaluate that development (Hammer et al. 2003). The addition of professional identify formation as a key aspect of a health professions student's transition into a practitioner creates another level of complexity as many educators struggle to see how these two formations differ and furthermore how to evaluate whether a learner has progressed. Chapter 8 in this book will examine both these roles and how they impact Millennials and Gen Z learners' transitions into health professionals.

CHAPTER SUMMARY AND CONCLUSION

Navigating multigenerational learners is an important aspect of the teaching and learning experience both for educators and learners. Gen Zs entry into higher education placed new expectations on faculty. While this generation shares similar learning preferences to Millennials, the level of engagement and hands-on learning expected by this cohort called for faculty to revitalize their curriculum. Understanding how to balance learning expectations in a multigenerational learning environment will be crucial to ensure that neither generation feels excluded or overlooked. However, this is only one piece of a much larger puzzle that encompasses how institutions of higher education function. In the next chapter, we explore recent trends impacting higher education across generations to include a look at the impact of declining college student enrollment, the demographic shifts of learners to include this impact on health professions education, and the evolving nature of student services and recruitment.

Chapter 3

Recent Trends Impacting Higher Education across Generations

Is Demography Destiny in Higher Education?

Given the unique qualities that each successive generation brings to bear, consideration of these qualities in the development and implementation of learning opportunities and support systems within institutions of higher education is needed. However, we must also recognize that there are considerable differences within these generational groups that should be acknowledged in order to tailor experiences to the unique needs of individuals. Still, recent and evolving trends in the demographics of college applicants have a significant impact on planning. These must be taken into account to ensure the effectiveness and viability of colleges and universities. This chapter will introduce and discuss those trends regarding numbers of applicants, race, ethnicity, gender, age, and trends in the use of technology and student preferences to paint a picture of the future of college enrollment and services in the decades to come.

SHIFTING GENERATIONS IN HIGHER EDUCATION

Millennials arrived on the higher education scene around the turn of the 21st century. They were known for prioritizing a solid sense of tradition and desire for community-building activities and more and different amenities on college campuses (Rickes 2016). Generation Z has begun to break with the Millennial generation in an effort to forge their own path. Given the four-fold cycle of generations, Rickes (2016) describes the Silent Generation as the historical analog to Gen Z, marked by an overprotective childhood, resulting in greater risk aversion and conformity compared to prior generations. Though they rely heavily on technology for work and school responsibilities, Gen Zs also have a propensity to gravitate toward pursuits that mimic the "good ole days" with a break from technology in their personal lives. This tendency is evidenced by the resurgence of vinyl record sales, tabletop games, and adult coloring books. These trends will bring a new set of expectations from prospective college students. With an increased focus by Generation Z on meaningful careers and employability, coupled with faster time-to-degree, colleges may shift their focus increasingly toward curriculum and delivery, technological skills, and continuous learning (Rickes 2016). The arrival of a new generation on college campuses is occurring alongside a shift in student demographics that has been expected for quite some time, with additional effects that were somewhat unexpected.

Father of sociology Auguste Comte is often attributed as saying, "Demography is destiny," with demography defined as the study of the composition, distinct characteristics, and trends in human populations. Though the true source of this quote is uncertain, and it may be somewhat of an overstatement, the question explored in this chapter is how shifting demography and related trends will affect the landscape of higher education in the coming decades. This chapter will review demographic trends that have shaped the "face" of college students across the United States and propose subsequent impacts on higher education and ways to address them.

FALLING OVER THE DEMOGRAPHIC CLIFF

Student enrollment in higher education has been impacted by multiple factors in the 2020s, which will have sustained effects into the 2030s and beyond. What has been described as a "demographic cliff" is expected to lead to a steady decline in the number of high school graduates, starting around 2026, with steep declines by 2029 as children of the Great Recession reach college age (Grawe 2018, 45). Referring to this period, which he describes as "demographic doldrums," Johnson proposes that "slight to modest" decreases in numbers of applicants are anticipated to affect a large number of colleges and universities (2019, 142). The threat of the demographic cliff occurs alongside a "systematic transfer of college operating costs to students," making robust enrollment critical to the financial stability of institutions of higher education (Harvey 2021, 3). Declining enrollment means financial trouble for institutions largely dependent on tuition dollars to sustain operations.

Grawe introduces the Higher Education Demand Index (HEDI) in his book *Demographics and the Demand for Higher Education* (2018). This index utilizes data from the 2002 Educational Longitudinal Study to predict the likelihood of college enrollment based on several demographic factors, including sex, race, ethnicity, parent education, geographic location, family income, family composition, and nativity. The HEDI differentiates projections based on institutional type (four-year or two-year institution), region, and prestige. Using this predictive modeling approach, Grawe projected as much as a 20% reduction in the pool of traditional first-year college students in some parts of the United States, with an 11% reduction on average across the nation (2018). He proposes that these shifts in demographics will likely affect institutions to varying degrees, depending on the institution type and region. Accounting for the probability of college attendance can actually reverse the effect of falling birth rates for some institutions. For example, regions with larger proportions of non-Hispanic whites, high-income families, and well-educated parents, such as the New England and Middle Atlantic regions, have historically had much higher rates of college enrollment compared to regions like the West South Central region, which has a higher proportion of Hispanic residents and those of lower socioeconomic status. Given these disparities, the market for college education may be thriving in some regions despite losses in population. Grawe goes on to explain that a demographic shift in the US population toward the Southeast can be attributed to immigration, interstate migration, and fertility differences among demographic groups, creating varying impacts across regions within the United States (2018). The next and subsequent sections will discuss how shifts in population and demographics may affect higher education.

Immigration, Migration, and Fertility as Factors Driving Shifts

Rates of immigration into the United States have remained relatively stable overall since the 1980s, with a brief spike after 1989 when the Immigration Reform and Control Act created a surge in immigration as amnesty provisions allowed previously undocumented immigrants to attain legal status, with rates that returned to prior levels by 1992 (Grawe 2018). Immigration into the United States directly alters the racial/ethnic distribution of the US population and subsequently indirectly affects future demand for higher education. The effect varies in different parts of the country due to uneven inflows across states, with certain cities seeing much larger numbers of immigrants because they are disembarkation points, creating a disproportionally higher impact in the Southwest and along the Atlantic coast (Grawe 2018).

Similarly, interstate migration can impact population distributions. Differential movement in and out of certain geographic regions in the United States can affect future markets for higher education. For example, there is evidence of migration of children out of the Pacific and mid-Atlantic regions of the country and into the South, potentially increasing the demand for higher education in this area of the country (Grawe 2018). Interstate migration can be influenced by the cost of living (particularly housing costs), job opportunities, quality of elementary and secondary schools, and safety, among other factors. According to North American Moving Services, Arizona, Tennessee, the Carolinas, Florida, and Texas were top destinations for movers (North American Moving Services 2021).

Demographic distribution across the United States can also be impacted by differing birth rates between population subgroups (Grawe 2018). For example, fertility rates, or rates of birth among women of reproductive age, among Hispanic and non-Hispanic black women have exceeded the national average over the past 25 years (Grawe 2018). However, an overall decreasing trend in fertility rates can obviously impact the demand for higher education downstream. Grawe refers to this situation as the "birth dearth" and details its potential impacts on college enrollment (2018, 12). Following a period of growth from the 1970s to 1990 and a relatively stable period for the next 15 years, the birth rate in the United States has continued to fall from its last peak in 2007 to a record low in 2020 (Hamilton, Martin, and Osterman 2021). This could negatively affect expected college enrollments into the 2030s. Notably, alongside this decline in birth rate, the death rate continues to climb, with 2021 recording the highest number of deaths in US history at the time of this publication, according to the Centers for Disease Control and Prevention National Center for Health Statistics (Ahmad and Cisewski 2022).

Work to model US birth rates based on historical data suggests that rates are not expected to rebound any time in the near future, potentially extending this estimate even further (Kearney and Levine 2021). According to available data as of 2018, though the number of students graduating from high school is expected to fall, there are also greater proportions of graduating seniors choosing to go to college (National Center for Higher Education Management Systems n.d.). However, this trend toward more students choosing a college education is not expected to overcome the previously mentioned factors impacting the number of enrollees, leaving colleges anxious about falling enrollment numbers. Accordingly, institutions of higher education will likely respond by recruiting more non-traditional students, leading to a shift in college student demographics and more diversity in generational cohort membership of enrollees.

SHIFTING DEMOGRAPHICS OF COLLEGE ENROLLEES

Students from across the Globe

International students have historically been drawn to the United States by the high quality of education and access to job opportunities post-graduation, with remarkable growth in international student enrollment since the 1950s (Institute of International Education [IIE] 2020). Enrollment of international students in the United States has great financial, cultural, and educational value, creating more tuition dollars, greater cultural diversity, and a better understanding of cultural differences, as well as initiation of lasting international collaborations (Johnson 2019). However, rising costs of higher education in the United States, high numbers of visa delays and denials, a challenging political environment, and expanded opportunities to study in other countries contributed to a marked decline in higher education enrollment by international students in the United States in the 2019–2020 academic year (Israel and Batalova 2021). Johnson (2019) discusses challenges in recruitment of international students, given the ever-changing US foreign policy and immigration laws, as well as rapid growth and strengthening quality of higher education in other parts of the world, such as China and India. A decline in the number of international enrollees can have a huge negative impact by decreasing cultural diversity of institutions of higher education (Jackson 2019). Colleges and universities will need to make concerted and targeted recruitment efforts to rebuild and sustain international student applications in order to thrive.

Shifts in Race and Ethnicity among Domestic College Applicants

Despite these negative impacts on international student enrollment, domestic college applicants are predicted to come from increasingly diverse racial and ethnic backgrounds in the coming decade. The applicant pool is expected to comprise relatively fewer white students and more Hispanic and Asian/Pacific Islander students (Johnson 2019). Further contributing to this trend is a rapid reduction in high school dropout rate among Hispanic students, from 34% in 1999 to 10% in 2016, a far greater decrease than that of black, white, or Asian students, as described by a report from the Pew Research Center (Gramlich 2017). The report notes that enrollment rates of Hispanic students in public and private colleges have increased 180% during that same period. Complicating this picture are the racial and ethnic disparities in degree completion, with lower completion rates among Hispanic and black students compared to Asian and white students, indicating a need not only for focused enrollment efforts but also for strategies to improve the retention of students from these population subgroups (Johnson 2019).

The College Enrollment Conundrum: Fewer Men Are Going to College

Another trend that institutions of higher education are grappling with is the decline in enrollment among men compared to women. Rates of college enrollment and completion among men have fallen precipitously in recent years, widening a gender gap that has been growing since the 1990s, and this phenomenon is happening globally (Reeves and Smith 2021). According to a report by the Chronicle for Higher Education, male undergraduate enrollment in the United States fell by 7% in fall 2020, almost three times that of female undergraduates (Field 2021b). Today, women account for 57% of college student enrollment (Field 2021b). Further magnifying the effect, of those students who enrolled in a four-year college in 2013, men were 10% less likely to graduate in four years compared to women (Reeves and Smith 2021). This trend is even more staggering among men of color attending community colleges (Robertson 2021). Robertson proposes potential reasons for the wide gender gap, including the assertion that boys in K–12 schools earn lower grades and spend less time studying compared to girls, and men have lower rates of college enrollment and drop out before graduation more often compared to women (2021).

Especially in communities of color, men are often expected to be providers, and going to college may be viewed as a waste of time and money (Field 2021b). In the face of the COVID-19 pandemic, men also felt more pressure to work as their family members lost jobs. However, the short-term economic gains of forgoing college could result in long-term losses, as the gap in earnings between men with high school diplomas and those with undergraduate college degrees has widened to more than $900,000 in median lifetime earnings (Field 2021b). Aside from the broad social and policy implications of having fewer men who are adequately prepared for the modern workforce, this gender gap can directly impact diversity in the college classroom (Stoet and Geary 2020). Programs specifically designed to address low retention rates and targeted at black male students are being adopted at multiple college campuses, attempting to reduce financial, academic, and social barriers in the early months of Freshman year (Robertson 2021). In addition, colleges are adding majors and sports teams that are more attractive to males (Field 2021b).

Rise of the Non-Traditional Student

The age distribution of students enrolling in institutions of higher education has also changed in the past several decades. According to the National Center for Education Statistics, enrollment of adults 35 years of age or older in degree-granting postsecondary institutions doubled from 1980 to 2019 and is projected to continue to hold steady into 2029; enrollment of full-time students in this age group quadrupled during the same period and is projected to grow (National Center for Education Statistics [NCES] 2020b). It is interesting to note that while this trend holds true for males, enrollment of females in this age group has remained steady and at higher numbers than that of males. Johnson proposes that these adult students, typically referred to as "non-traditional," are becoming the "new traditional student," making this group the largest student population on many college campuses (2019, 47). Bernhard describes the rapid growth in numbers of students over the age of 40 enrolling in college as an "imperative pursuit" and attributes this trend to layoffs, divorce, unfulfilled career goals, and lack of opportunity for career growth in their current industry as drivers of this trend (2020, 34).

Johnson describes the unique challenges faced by non-traditional students (2019). They often have full-time employment and need class schedules that accommodate working hours. They may travel greater distances to campus, further affecting schedules as well as expenses. A large proportion are married or divorced, and many are parents, some being single parents. These non-traditional students often have different health statuses and healthcare needs, and they may have very limited time to participate in social events or campus activities. In addition to these individual barriers encountered by non-traditional students, institutional barriers also exist, including stigma toward older learners, lack of recognition of credentials and prior learning, and difficulty obtaining financial aid (Johnson 2019).

Amenities and services on college campuses often miss the mark on meeting the needs of this unique population. This noteworthy shift in the age of students enrolling in postsecondary institutions means that, while Gen Z will become a focus in regard to characteristics and learning styles, the needs of Millennial learners, as well as those from prior generations, will still be an important focus, and teaching faculty will be challenged with effectively delivering content in ways that both Gen Z and Millennials desire. Subsequent chapters in this book will delve deeper into this conundrum.

In the face of these changing demographics, institutes of higher education will need to be nimble in responding to the needs of a diverse student population. A greater emphasis on the recruitment of minority and first-generation students will be necessary while also strengthening efforts to retain students from these more financially vulnerable populations. Students from low-income families tend to seek college loans in greater amounts and have higher dropout rates compared to students from upper-income families (Johnson 2019). Of note, almost a third of American students who take out loans to attend college never complete their degree, and students from low-income families who take out large loans and never finish college often find it extremely challenging to pay them off (Johnson 2019). Given the demographic phenomena and resulting challenges described above, university leaders will need to holistically reassess policies, procedures, practices, and budgets. Health professions programs will need to be particularly aware of and ready for these challenges.

DEMOGRAPHIC TRENDS SPECIFIC TO HEALTH PROFESSIONS EDUCATION

The gender, racial, and ethnic diversity, as well as the age of health professions students are continuously evolving. An examination of gender, race, and ethnicity of students enrolled in medical school from 1978 to 2019 using data provided by the Association of American Medical Colleges revealed stark differences in gender distribution over that period, with a much larger proportion of men enrolling compared to women in 1978 (by a factor of three) but steady decreases in the men to women ratio over time (Morris et al. 2021). By 2019, medical schools seem to have attained gender parity, with the percentage of female medical students (50.6%) slightly surpassing that of males. An even more striking trend has been observed in veterinary schools, with a shift from 11% female enrollment in 1970 to just over 80% in 2017 (American Association of Veterinary Medical Colleges [AAVMC] 2023). According to the American Association of Colleges of Nursing, the percentage of graduates who are male ranged from 11.4% to 14.3% in 2022, depending on the program (American Association of Colleges of Nursing [AACN] 2023).

With an increasingly diverse US patient population, a more diverse healthcare professions workforce is greatly needed. The National Academy of Medicine stresses that increasing diversity among healthcare professionals improves access to care for racial and ethnic minorities (Institute of Medicine 2004). Wilbur et al. assert that while racial and ethnic diversity has increased in the United States with an expectation that racial and ethnic minorities will make up the majority of the US population by 2043, diversity in many health professions has not kept pace (2020). Though the overall healthcare workforce is more diverse than the general US population, the majority of people of color in the healthcare workforce are in lower-paying or entry-level positions without much opportunity for advancement (Wilbur et al. 2020).

Although diversity among college students has recently increased, as discussed earlier in this chapter, people of color are still underrepresented among students enrolled in health professions programs. More specifically, Morris et al. found that though the proportion of Asian medical students increased from 1978 to 2019, progress in increasing representation among other racial and ethnic minority groups has been very slow (2021). In 2023, approximately 80% of students enrolled in colleges of veterinarian medicine were white (AAVMC 2023). In contrast, 43% of undergraduate enrollees in nursing programs were from racial and ethnic minorities, with slightly lower percentages (35.8–40.7%) across the different nursing graduate programs (AACN 2023). Health professions programs will need to continue to find ways to recruit and retain people of color through targeted recruitment and the creation of programs to better meet their needs.

The directionality of trends in the age of health professions students has been mixed across professions. Between 2014 and 2018, the average age of matriculated medical students held steady at 24 years (Association of American Medical Colleges 2017). Age-related data are no longer reported by this organization as of 2019. The percentage of graduating student pharmacists who were 25 years of age or under has decreased steadily from 49.4% in 2012 to 41.8% in 2021, and the percentage of graduating student pharmacists 26 to 30 years of age has increased from 37.3% to 42.1%, indicating an upward shift in mean age (American Association of Colleges of Pharmacy n.d.). The increase in mean age of pharmacy school graduates since the early 2000s is likely due in part to a shift from pharmacy programs awarding mostly bachelor's degrees to programs offering only doctoral degrees, which typically take at least a year longer to complete. Likewise, prerequisite requirements have expanded over that period such that many students entering pharmacy programs have already earned a four-year degree prior to admission.

For nursing education programs, the average age of students in professional programs has oscillated. The AACN no longer tracks the age of nursing students and, as such, makes determining the demographic trend of this profession challenging. However, the Texas Center for Nursing Workforce Studies found that in 2013, the largest proportion of students (43.7%) newly enrolled in a registered nursing (RN) program in Texas were between 26 and 40 years of age, with 37.2% between ages 21 and 25 and only 8.2% in the under-21 age group (Texas Center for Nursing Workforce Studies, 2022). By 2016, there was a shift, with 13.4% in the under-21 age group. The largest proportion (39.4%) were between 21 and 25 years of age, and a similar proportion (38.1%) were in the 26–40 age group. In 2021, the latest available data, the largest proportion (37%) was again in the 26–40 age group, a similar proportion (36%) in the 21–25 age group, and 18.7% in the under-21 age group.

In veterinary medicine, applicants in the 25–30 age group represented only 16% of the total applicant pool in 2013, with 21- and 22-year-olds representing the greatest proportion (28% and 19%, respectively; AAVMC 2023). In contrast, the average age for first-year veterinary medicine program enrollees was 23.3 years in 2016. This shift may be due to the competitive qualifications of program applicants seeking to gain more educational experience prior to applying. Age data is not available for other years from this source.

ENTER THE COVID-19 PANDEMIC

All of this uncertainty was compounded exponentially when COVID-19 came onto the scene in early 2020. In addition to the previously discussed factors negatively affecting enrollment in institutions of higher education in the United States over the last couple of decades, a precipitous 8% drop in enrollment was seen between 2019 and 2022, presumably due to the pandemic (National Student Clearinghouse Research Center [NSCRC] 2022a). The abrupt, unexpected, and extensive changes brought about by the pandemic, including but not limited to the transition to remote operations and subsequent online learning modalities, made it abundantly clear that dramatic shifts in the operations of institutes of higher education are possible and sometimes necessary. Unfortunately, the "baby bump" that was speculated to occur in light of the stay-at-home orders early in the pandemic did not seem to transpire, and the contraction in the pool of high school graduates bound for college is expected to continue until at least 2039 (Harvey 2021).

The immigration policy landscape was also volatile and confusing amid the COVID-19 pandemic, with an initial attempt to bar international students from entering or remaining in the United States if schools offered only online coursework (Israel and Batalova 2021). Although this attempt was quickly quashed, schools took a reactive stance to try to protect students against any similar attempts in the future. For example, some universities enrolled international students in research credit courses for a minimum of one credit hour to meet the requirement of less than 100% of credit hours being in online courses. This and other policy barriers added to the uncertainty and hesitation of prospective students, further impacting enrollment into fall 2020.

The pandemic has brought with it increased emotional stress, financial concerns, and tensions surrounding social injustice and issues of diversity, equity, and inclusion; and these factors have impacted students' views on attending college and the variables they consider when selecting an institution for higher education. Many students decided to take a gap year, and some of those may not return to college post-pandemic. Those who are enrolling are carefully evaluating institutions' efforts to safeguard student safety through pandemic restrictions, with some highly valuing these efforts and others choosing to avoid those institutions that have stricter guidelines, such as social distancing and more remote learning (Selingo 2021). Likewise, many students are seeking institutions with easy-to-access and well-resourced services to support mental health. This is of particular concern among Gen Z learners. Services to support both mental health and disabilities among students will continue to be a focus. Institutions' social culture, including their stance on issues of diversity, equity, and inclusion and their policies against social injustice, are becoming important factors of consideration to student applicants. In addition, many institutions are shifting their policies related to standardized testing requirements upon application, impacting student decision making. The next section will further explore how these demographic shifts and recent changes in focus may impact campus services.

IMPACT OF A SHIFTING COLLEGE DEMOGRAPHIC ON CAMPUS SERVICES

Prompted by the COVID-19 pandemic and other factors, there has been a continued rise in consumerism among college students, and institutions are following suit to meet the ever-changing demands of their primary customers (Plunkett 2014). From what we know about Generation Z, they desire only those elements of a college experience that serve the purpose of preparing them for a successful career, and they want to graduate in as little time as possible. This laser focus on navigating college will have enormous effects on the demand for campus services and the structure and function in which they serve. The price of obtaining a college degree has risen steeply over the past 40 years. This is driven by (1) lagging effects of fee increases as compared to rising cost per student resulting in stagnant productivity, (2) increasing cost of hiring a highly educated workforce, and (3) rising standards of care in education (Archibald and Feldman 2018). With the increasing cost of education comes greater and more specific demand from consumers, leading faculty and administrators into a position in which they feel they must cater to the students' every request. Plunkett states, "The unfortunate reaction to the Student Consumerism behaviors from many postsecondary educators is fear and obsequiousness to the requests and demands of the student" (2014, 2).

For Gen Z learners, institutions will need to revisit fee structures and campus amenities to better meet their demands. This generation prefers to only utilize the services they really need and will, therefore, want to pay fees for services à la carte. This will undoubtedly have substantial impacts on budgets, especially at institutions that rely heavily on revenue from student fees. In addition to restructuring services, utilization of campus study and workspace is likely to change. With increasing reliance on and comfort with technology and, accordingly, a growing trend of remote work, students, faculty, and staff are less likely to utilize traditional work and study spaces on campus. As described in a report published by Microsoft (2021), a study that analyzed LinkedIn profiles of hundreds of millions of members found that Gen Z employees were more likely to apply for remote work positions (21%) compared to employees of older generations (18%). Gen Z employees also indicated that they are struggling more with feeling engaged and excited about work post-pandemic compared to older generations.

Already widely used by technology firms, an evolving trend in office space management in the post-COVID-19 environment of hybrid work is the use of "hoteling spaces," or shared office space that employees reserve when they want to work on-site (Dickler 2021). This trend is likely to spread to college campuses as facilities management strives for more efficient and cost-effective use of space in campus buildings. A benefit of hoteling spaces, aside from cost savings in reduction of square footage and accordingly reduced use of utilities, is that they are more conducive to teamwork and collaboration compared to traditional office and study spaces. However, some argue that the productivity of knowledge workers can be negatively impacted by such working environments that do not allow for long periods of focused, uninterrupted time (Newport 2018). There is no doubt that the COVID-19 pandemic will have a lasting impact on how businesses operate, and this will also apply to institutions of higher education. A good example of the effect of the pandemic on how educational programs operate is the broadening scope of learning approaches delivered online.

RISE OF ONLINE LEARNING (CULTURE EATS TECHNOLOGY FOR BREAKFAST)

Despite falling numbers of college applicants, as noted above, enrollment in online programs continues to increase (Schroeder 2021). In the face of the COVID-19 pandemic, the number of undergraduate students enrolled in exclusively online programs increased by more than 350%, and growth at public four-year institutions was 2–3 times higher than rates at private nonprofit institutions (Lederman 2021). According to a survey of colleges and universities, 59% reported that they "plan to continue some or all of their emergency remote learning offerings via distance education after the pandemic" (Lederman 2021).

Adult students value the flexibility and accessibility of online learning. With the increase in adults returning to college while maintaining employment, this flexibility will be a major factor in the choice of institution.

Regarding Millennial and Gen Z learners, given their propensity to embrace and even prefer the use of technology, the provision of online learning in this group could present fewer challenges than learners from older generations. However, as mentioned in Chapter 5, Gen Z tends to prefer face-to-face or blended instruction more so than Millennials. Even so, institutions of higher education will need to strongly consider the expansion of online programs in order to meet the needs for flexibility and accessibility voiced as critical by students of multiple generations.

An Educause showcase series titled "The Digital versus Brick-and-Mortar Balancing Game" proposes that "culture eats technology for breakfast" (Educause n.d., para 2). Innovative technologies are no doubt needed to address the needs of a new generation of learners with the expansion of online and hybrid (combination of online and on-site) courses, but without the necessary culture shifts, faculty, and administrators at institutions of higher education may not embrace this high-tech vision of the classroom of the future. These culture shifts include remote work, skills-based learning, cybersecurity concerns, sustainability, and the value of a degree. Professional development for these teaching modalities has a high degree of potential impact on learning outcomes, with relatively low requirements for new literacies, according to the report. Transformation and redesign of physical learning spaces to create inclusive classrooms for hybrid learning will allow both faculty and students to benefit, but this will require overcoming some significant hurdles. The hesitation to move to hybrid or online learning models is deeply rooted among many more traditional faculty members. Finding ways to eliminate the stereotype of online learning and rally buy-in from faculty and staff will be a much-needed focus for institutions of higher education as we move through (and beyond) the information age (Birkenshaw n.d.).

Online Learning in the Health Professions

Health professions education is not immune to these shifts toward online learning. In a DigiMed study, medical students who were surveyed from twelve different countries mostly embraced the shift to online learning that occurred in response to the pandemic (Stoehr et al. 2021). They indicated that this modality offered greater flexibility during the pandemic without reducing attendance. A large majority (78%) of respondents indicated that medical education lags behind the current capabilities of online learning (Stoehr et al. 2021). They preferred a more balanced offering of online versus on-site learning, with at least 40% of content offered online, compared to 14% pre-pandemic. Students displayed a high degree of intrinsic motivation and a willingness to invest in technology to support their learning in an online environment. Stoehr and colleagues propose that the difficulty students faced with lack of motivation to complete online modules may be due more to the type of content (e.g., lecture-based versus problem-based) rather than the format of delivery (online versus on-site) (2021). Educators will need to be trained in the delivery of effective pedagogy that lends itself to impactful online learning to stay relevant in an increasingly digital world.

Online learning for health professions has several benefits, including allowing clinicians who currently work to continue to do so while pursuing further education in the health professions. The digital format also allows for innovation in teaching, such as simulations of virtual patients and the use of immersive technologies. Stoehr and colleagues also propose that the increased flexibility of online learning may address issues of student diversity and inclusivity in health professions education (2021). Downsides to online learning that must also be considered are social isolation of students, less direct interaction with instructors, and blurred lines between work and home environments, leading to difficulty stepping away from work to attend to personal responsibilities. Rather than emergency measures to shift quickly to online learning that were necessary with the COVID-19 pandemic, a curricular framework based on a thoughtfully designed model of blended or hybrid learning using an evidence-based approach may be an effective path forward for health professions education.

THE EVOLVING FACE OF RECRUITMENT

In addition to changes in how programs utilize technology to shape the learning experience, the trends previously discussed may have a significant impact on student recruitment. With changes in the demographics of individuals seeking a college education, institutions of higher education will need to be proactive in their approach to recruiting. Student services to meet the needs of an increasingly diverse student population will be a critical factor. Focusing specifically on Gen Z students, recruitment efforts will need to consider the unique characteristics of this new generation of applicants while continuing to meet the needs of Millennial learners and older generations.

When considering college selection, price is a significant factor in choosing a school for Gen Z students more so than Millennials, with many favoring in-state programs due to cost savings. Parents tend to play a significant role in college attendance and selection decisions, with Gen Z students seeking substantial input from their parents. For this reason, engaging parents by providing resources, open lines of communication, and educational sessions specifically for parents are approaches that many institutions are taking to enhance recruitment and retention of students. (Field et al. 2021). In addition, many Gen Z learners forgo residential living, opting to live at home in order to budget for college tuition and expenses, in stark contrast to Millennials. It is expected that Gen Zs will also favor living at home after graduation while they save money and pay off loans in anticipation of purchasing a home, particularly in the face of rising housing prices (Federal Reserve Economic Database 2023). They also have shortened the time spent in college by dedicating themselves to a career path earlier than prior generations, who tended to place more value on the college journey (Seemiller and Grace 2019a). Alternative schooling options, like community colleges and massive open online courses, have enticed Gen Z learners due to the cost savings they promote.

Gen Zs tend to be hard-working, with 55% of high school seniors in 2016 willing to work overtime to do a good job, in contrast with 44% of Millennial high school seniors in 2004, according to a piece published on the website for Comeveo, a software company serving institutions of higher education (Comeveo 2018). They are quite averse to incurring student loan debt, with 66% indicating this as their top concern. Gen Z students, being digital natives, communicate entirely through their screens and rely heavily on internet research to compare value among different institutions of higher education. In regard to communication preferences, Gen Zs are amenable to sharing personal information and prefer that organizations tailor communication to them personally, which suggests that colleges should utilize this strategy for effective recruitment.

Gen Z spends more time on their smartphones than their laptops, so designing mobile content is critical to effective recruitment for this population. Video content is a favorite of this generation, with 70% reporting they watch YouTube an average of two hours per day (Comeveo 2018). Many institutions have developed applications for recruitment purposes, and in-app notifications can be very effective among this population to notify them of events on campus or new content (Comeveo 2018). Authenticity and transparency are of utmost importance to this generation. Content targeted to specific groups and tailored to students' personal experiences are among their stated preferences. With the propensity to use social media and subsequent importance placed on peer influences among Gen Z, colleges have turned to strategies such as peer-to-peer recruiting using platforms like Skype and FaceTime to connect potential students with current students to ask about campus amenities, culture, academics, and college life. Student testimonials and blogs can also be effective for this purpose. With an average attention span of 8 minutes, Gen Z will require content to be short and to the point (Comeveo 2018).

As mentioned earlier, Gen Zs and Millennials are driven by purpose and values and tend to be more global-minded than previous generations. Therefore, colleges will need to meet these needs by advertising their commitment to issues such as environment, justice, diversity, equity, and inclusion and its impact on the broader community. Being very practical, Gen Z will be attracted to institutions of higher education based on value rather than frills. They will prefer to utilize only those student services they see as benefiting them in their pursuit of a successful career, so recruitment will need to highlight the return on investment or value for their tuition dollars. While it will be critical to consider the unique demands of Gen Z recruits, given the upward shifts in age in many educational programs, institutions will still need to consider the wants and needs of Millennials who may make up a large proportion of non-traditional students when planning recruitment efforts.

The 2023 landmark decision by the Supreme Court of the United States has altered how colleges can use targeted enrollment practices to diversify the student population based on race, ethnicity, and national origin (Chamberlain 2023). However, this ruling places no stipulations on recruitment of or outreach to diverse populations. Given this outcome, a reexamination of recruitment best practices will be crucial to support ongoing efforts to engage students from diverse backgrounds regarding the value of attending the institution.

IMPACTS ON GRADUATE EDUCATION POST-PANDEMIC

In addition to the effects on various aspects of undergraduate education, recent trends have also impacted graduate programs. Certainly, anything that negatively impacts undergraduate enrollment is expected to have trickle-down effects on enrollment in graduate programs, and the trends noted above are expected to have an impact on programs beginning around 2030. Interestingly, enrollment in graduate programs has actually increased since 2019 by 4.9%, but growth may have been stifled by the pandemic (NSCRC 2022a), and it is difficult to say how this growth is expected to be impacted by 2030. In addition to these, other factors are at play that can further influence graduate program enrollment, such as fluctuating immigration policies and changes in standardized testing requirements. The unstable political landscape leading up to and coinciding with the COVID-19 pandemic in the United States created constantly changing policies related to immigration. This uncertainty for potential international students was compounded by the fear of contracting the virus during the height of the pandemic and hesitation to engage in remote learning modalities. Because many graduate programs in the United States rely heavily on international applicants, the impacts of the pandemic were far-reaching (Fischer 2021). Many prospective international students preferred to delay application or defer offers of admission rather than participate remotely online or in a hybrid modality. Related, greater obstacles to application and immigration, along with mounting political tension, have led to fewer applications received from countries like China and India, which have historically supplied a large portion of international graduate students in the United States (Fischer 2021).

Further affecting graduate program admissions processes, waivers for requirements related to standardized test scores occurred when access to testing was severely limited due to worldwide shutdowns during the height of the pandemic. This has prompted programs to rethink these requirements going forward, considering the already existing debate about the equity and validity of standardized tests for admissions considerations (Kent and McCarthy 2016). Many programs have adopted a permanent halt to the requirement for standardized test scores and are moving to a more holistic approach to admissions considerations. While this has created opportunities for enrollment where they previously may not have existed, programs have struggled to find alternative metrics to evaluate candidates' academic promise, thinking and problem-solving skills, and social competence. As for graduate programs as a whole, there have also been impacts on workforce development, explored in the next section.

CHANGING WORKFORCE

A similar shift in the higher education landscape is the evolution of the workforce, discussed further in Chapter 10 of this book. Holzer (2015) recognizes a decline in well-paid clerical, construction, and production jobs often filled by high school graduates. In juxtaposition to this trend, he describes a shift in the middle-wage job market with a rise in areas that require more postsecondary education or training, including health technology, information technology, advanced manufacturing, and various service jobs, labeling this sector as the "newer middle" (Holzer 2015, 1). In addition, the demand for skills in formerly low-skill jobs is increasing. Holzer goes on to explain that filling these "newer middle" positions has proved difficult for employers faced with impending retirement from their Baby Boomer employees and proposes that employers look to institutions of higher education to better prepare and cultivate a new group of workers to fill these positions (2015, 1).

To fill this role, these institutions will need policy changes that provide more support and incentives for training and skill development for this group of future workers. Federal funding has historically supported these programs, but dropout rates are high, and graduates sometimes complete the training without the credentials that are valued by the labor market. To partially address this issue, new collaborations are being built between industry and institutions of higher education. One such approach is known as sectoral training, with partnerships between training providers, typically community colleges, and employers to ensure that proper training is delivered, with the commitment to hiring those trainees once their training is completed. Career pathways is a similar approach that combines didactic training with real-world experience. These programs have demonstrated large positive impacts on earnings for the working poor (Holzer 2015). Still, the quality of such programs is difficult to replicate and maintain, and low-income workers may lack basic academic skills in areas such as science, technology, engineering, and mathematics (STEM) fields that equip them for proper technical training.

Community and lower-tiered four-year colleges often lack the resources to produce high-quality learning options and the needed career counseling services to prepare students for the job market. Holzer suggests that more incentives for these institutions are needed to help fill this gap (2015). He strongly advocates broad policy proposals to create incentive systems and funding for institutions of higher education to build relevant skills and improve the preparedness of students in ways that the labor market will reward. This should include multiple components. More resources and better incentives for public colleges are needed. High-quality career and technical education (historically known as vocational education in the United States) should be supported. Employers should be encouraged to create more good jobs. Lastly, other supportive policies and practices are needed, such as increases in the minimum wage, paid leave for all workers, and allowing for the formation of "working councils" at non-union firms to give employees a voice in decisions made by management (Holzer 2015, 7).

Got Skills?

Additionally, changing workforce environments and opportunities are leading more college graduates to return to college for reskilling and upskilling, leading to the expansion of credentialing and certificate programs, which provide opportunities for career advancement in less time and at a lower cost (Schroeder 2021). Reskilling is defined as training workers to develop new skills and competencies that will allow them to change to a completely new occupation, while upskilling is defined as training to develop new skills to optimize performance in their current occupation (US Office of Personnel Management 2019). Paullet, Behling, and Behling (2020) discuss higher education's expanding role in reskilling and upskilling, describing a situation in which large numbers of jobs are being created, but the number of qualified workers is falling, creating skills gaps in the workforce. Organizations are investing significant resources in reskilling and upskilling existing workers to bolster productivity, a more cost-effective approach than relying on new hires to fill these gaps (Paullet, Behling, and Behling 2020). This trend creates a need for institutions of higher education to cater to students who are older and may be returning to college through badges, credentials, certifications, and degree programs. Adult learners look for key features in a program, including time to completion, fit with their current lifestyle and family situation, and value that cannot be obtained elsewhere, and these factors may facilitate the rise in master's degree programs and stackable certificates that will attract adult learners (Bhushan et al. 2022).

Paullet, Behling, and Behling (2020) propose that developing and maintaining faculty skills and state-of-the-art knowledge to support reskilling and upskilling will be a significant challenge. These authors suggest strategies such as incentives, supportive training programs, and collaborations with businesses and industries to address this. They also suggest that course design for the purposes of reskilling and upskilling incorporates exploration, scaffolding, and higher-order thinking (analysis, evaluation, and synthesis) to better support working professionals. Lastly, they recommend that institutions of higher education invest in the recruitment of appropriate faculty, provision of adequate learning resources, and design of appropriate student support services that cater to a widening demographic.

CHAPTER SUMMARY AND CONCLUSION

This chapter reviews the influence of the "birth dearth," as well as shifting immigration and migration patterns, on student enrollment in institutes of higher education and how these institutions are likely to react to these trends (Grawe 2018, 12). Also discussed are the ways newer generations are constantly shaping the landscape of higher education in regard to structure and services, while older generations still need to be considered. Institutions will need to be nimble as they respond to these patterns in order to continue to thrive, particularly in the health professions.

Delving deeper into the factors that affect health professions education, Chapter 4 examines these factors in two broad categories, mental health, and the cost of education, in the context of Millennial and Gen Z learners. It will also provide guidance for educators and institutions to support mental health, increase enrollment, and manage costs.

Chapter 4

Factors That Impact Health Professions Education

Societal factors impacting Gen Zs' and Millennials' college experiences are immense and evolving. More than previous generations, including Millennials, Gen Zs place distinct value on prioritizing mental health, social awareness, and diversity (Gaspar and Waxer n.d.). As a result, mental health and well-being remain central to the Gen Z experience considering the traumatic events they collectively experienced at the turn of the 21st century and beyond (e.g., September 11th terror attacks, economic crises, and the COVID-19 pandemic). This chapter will focus on two key factors that impact the college experience for Gen Z and Millennial learners: (1) mental health awareness, including drug and alcohol use, and (2) college enrollment, including the cost of higher education. Recommendations to better support students in these two areas are embedded after both sections.

MENTAL HEALTH AWARENESS AND SUBSTANCE USE

The first factor impacting higher education relates to mental health awareness and substance use and abuse among Gen Zs and Millennials. Mental health issues are prevalent among college students (Pedrelli et al. 2015), as well as students in health professions (Dyrbye et al. 2008; Dyrbye et al. 2011). College presidents deem mental health concerns as one of the most critical issues on campus, not just because of the prevalence but also because students with unresolved mental health challenges are more likely to drop out of college (Field 2021a). In a national study conducted among college-aged students in 2020, 35% of respondents met the diagnostic criteria for major depressive disorder (MDD) and 39% met the diagnostic criteria for generalized anxiety disorder (GAD) (Soria and Horgos 2021). To a degree, this prevalence is not surprising given the digital propensity of Gen Zs and Millennials, and the social isolation that accompanies frequent use of digital devices and social media. Pfeifer et al. (2022) studied perceptions of stress among health professions students and found that when perceived stress increased, perceived anxiety increased as well. Correspondingly, students perceived emotional and social wellness decreased as a result.

Research shows that Gen Zs are more academically prepared than previous generations but struggle with essential life skills like coping, resilience, and time management (Kubaryk 2020a). In response, higher education programs have been brainstorming and implementing measures to mitigate mental health challenges by expanding counseling services, enhancing well-being initiatives, modifying grading to reduce anxiety, and teaching coping behaviors (MacPhee et al. 2021; Reed et al. 2011; Shiralkar et al. 2013). Despite these initiatives, it is important for institutions to have coordinated and focused initiatives that support mental health and well-being.

There are multiple national organizations that promote mental health awareness in the United States. Some organizations advocate and normalize mental health challenges, while others collect and summarize data on mental health trends. Examples of such organizations include the National Alliance on Mental Illness (NAMI), the Centers for Disease Control (CDC), Substance Abuse and Mental Health Services Administration (SAMHSA), and the Healthy Minds Study. A key statistic that should drive college educators is the prevalence of US college-aged students, which includes Millennials and Gen Zs, who experienced some form of mental illness: 1 in 3 young adults aged 18–25 years experienced some form of mental illness in 2020; whereas 1 in 10 experienced a "serious" mental illness (NAMI n.d.). Of the diagnosed mental illnesses in college-aged students, depression was the most common followed by anxiety (The Healthy Minds Study 2021). Vermeulen (2021) offered insight into the key concerns and anxieties of young adults: impact of politics on daily life; relationships with friends/family/colleagues; personal health; keeping yourself and your family safe; and finances, bills, and expenses. This indicates that young adults are experiencing mental health issues that stem from an assortment of factors.

The strain of navigating the transition to adulthood and experiencing adulthood stress for the first time can take its toll on the mental health of young adults. The Association for University and College Counseling Center Directors collects annual data on college and university counseling centers. Data from 2020 states that the most frequent mental health concern among college students who seek counseling services is anxiety, followed by depression, stress, and relational problems (LeViness et al. 2019). Gen Zs, however, have been shown to be hesitant to seek mental health counseling. For example, almost 90% of centers reported a 12.2% increase in demand for counseling services in 2019 as compared to 2018 (LeViness et al. 2019). The demand for counseling services is high and continues to rise. This could be in part due to the reduction in stigma associated with mental health treatment or the increase in prevalence of mental health conditions in current student populations. The data also indicates that college females are almost twice as likely to seek counseling services than their male peers. Students value counseling services, reporting that they are effective in improving retention and academic performance. Interestingly, almost 50% of counseling service centers are not integrated with any other office on campus, and much less across units at institutions (LeViness et al. 2019). If counseling services are embedded within a unit on campus, it is most likely to be within a specific school or college at the university. This is an interesting observation as universities are considering how to transition to a more comprehensive and coordinated approach to mental health support.

The prevalence of mental illness should be impressed upon college educators. If one in three students experience or has experienced a mental illness, the need to recognize the signs, symptoms, and strains associated with mental health concerns is crucial. It is also important to be able to act, intervene, and/or refer confidently. Results from Soria and Horgos (2021) indicate that students who are the greatest risk for developing MDD and GAD include those who identified as queer, gender non-binary, white or Asian, caregivers, having a disability, food, or housing insecure, experiencing financial strain or academic obstacles. On the other hand, those at lower risk of MDD or GAD were cisgender men, socioeconomically advantaged, straight, confident in sense of belonging, feeling valued and supported at the institution, and having a safe environment Soria and Horgos (2021).

Even if students have not been diagnosed with a mental illness, general mental health and well-being affects all students on campus. For institutions, there is not a single best approach to supporting students as it pertains to their mental health (Soria and Horgos 2021). Unfortunately, despite the breadth, support for mental health is given less attention than other factors affecting students, such as financial concerns, retention, social connectedness, belonging, and so on. (Lipson et al. 2019).

Substance Use and Abuse

Given the relevance of mental health concerns among Gen Z and Millennial college students, the prevalence of substance use and abuse is an important consideration. Substance abuse and mental illness are positively correlated. Individuals with a diagnosed mental illness were more likely to use illicit drugs than those without mental illness (Mental Health by the Numbers n.d.; SAMHSA 2020). The National Survey on Drug Use and Health is a survey conducted on behalf of SAMHSA, which is a program under the US

Department of Health and Human Services. This survey sheds light on the significant impact that substance abuse and mental health issues have on individuals, families, communities, and societies (SAMHSA 2020). A key finding from the 2020 report indicates the prevalence of substance abuse among those 12 years or older: almost 60% used tobacco, alcohol, or an illicit drug in the past month. Marijuana was the most commonly used illicit drug with almost 18% of people aged 12 years or older having used it in the past year. Despite the ubiquitous use of tobacco, alcohol, and illicit drug use, the majority of survey respondents recognize the harm associated with the use of these substances.

Drug use and abuse also involves prescription medications. In a robust study from 2012, researchers from the National Center for Health Statistics evaluated the prevalence of psychotropic medications in youth aged 12–17. Results indicated that approximately 6.6% of adolescents had used a psychotropic drug in the past month, with medications for treatment of attention deficit hyperactive disorder (ADHD) and depression being the most prevalent drug classes prescribed (Jonas 2013). The timing of this study is important because it coincides with the coming of age for Millennials and Generation Z. Interestingly, females of this age were more likely to use antidepressants while males were more likely to utilize ADHD medications.

While trends around mental health might be concerning, it has been getting the attention of US colleges and universities since Gen Zs have been coming of age. Renewed focus is being placed on meeting students' mental health needs, not just for the benefit of the students, but also because of the campus-wide benefit. Reducing depression in students benefits the entire campus in ways such as increasing student satisfaction, retention, individuals' lifetime earnings, institutional reputation, alumni donations, and societal benefits (Eisenberg, Golberstein, and Hunt 2009). To assist campus leaders in advocating for resources around mental health, a return-on-investment calculator was created to demonstrate the economic impact of investing in student mental health. It is based on population size, retention rate, and prevalence of depression. The calculator can be found at healthymindsnetwork.org.

Burnout

In addition to the mental health concerns and substance use/abuse, health professions students may be particularly susceptible to the occurrence of burnout (National Academies of Sciences, Engineering, and Medicine 2019). These students must learn to exist and interact within a variety of settings, both classroom and experiential. Unfortunately, conflicting demands can lead to a sense of stress, overwhelm, and/or burnout. The authors estimated that around one-third of medical students had experienced depersonalization, over one-third had experienced emotional exhaustion, and approximately half had experienced some degree of burnout. Burnout brings about many consequences for students in healthcare education fields, including lower levels of patient care quality, decreased ability to retain and apply knowledge, and decreased motivation for one's work (National Academies of Sciences, Engineering, and Medicine 2019).

Recommendations to Support Student Mental Health

Strategies for educators and institutions to better support current and future students regarding their mental health have been suggested. Before taking action, the American Council on Education proposes that institutions first assess student needs and available mental health resources in order to identify gaps (Lipson et al. 2019). This can be done through a systematic survey or informally through dialoguing with stakeholders. Once gaps are identified, focused plans can be created. Potential actions that colleges and universities can take to prioritize student mental health include the following:

1. Empowering educators with knowledge through professional development initiatives. This training might include signs of distress, student resources, and mental health first aid (Active Minds 2020; Field 2021a; Lipson et al. 2019).
2. Enhancing the accessibility of clinical services, which might include addressing cost, increasing sites, enhancing the range of services, and/or increasing appointment availabilities (Lipson et al. 2019).
3. Removing stigma by norm setting. In other words, normalize the need for help (Active Minds 2020). This might be done through marketing and enhancing communication around available mental health services provided on campus. Aiding this might also be health promotion and awareness programs across campus (Lipson et al. 2019).
4. Strengthening peer support structures, so students can better support one another (Field 2021a).
5. Adding trigger or content warnings for educational materials that might cause psychological distress (Plochocki 2019). This is especially pertinent within health professions education as students are taught about mental health disorders and their associated treatments. While this content might enhance one's understanding of issues that cause psychological distress, it might also be triggering for others.
6. Encouraging well-being practices within courses to mitigate burnout. This might include reasonable assignment deadlines, meditation during class, self-care as homework, and the practice of personal self-care as an example to students (Active Minds 2020).

7. Focusing on campus-wide well-being initiatives that promote student success, coping, and resilience (Kubaryk 2020b).
8. Cultivating a sense of belonging among students, as it serves as a protective factor against depression and anxiety (especially for underrepresented, first-generation, and first-year students) (Gopalan, Linden-Carmichael, and Lanza 2022).

Enhancing student mental health has positive effects across campus, including improved academic performance, persistence, and graduation rates (Lipson et al. 2019). Thus, investing in student mental health promotes a thriving academic and economic institution.

COLLEGE ENROLLMENT AND COST

The United States experienced a sharp incline in college enrollment post-9/11 (i.e., 2000–2010), which was a time when Millennial students were going to college (Hanson 2022; US Department of Education 2022). The increase in enrollment during this time was evident for both undergraduate and graduate programs. However, since 2010, undergraduate enrollment has been on a decline and universities have been struggling to meet their enrollment goals (Hanson 2022). As previously discussed in Chapter 3, the COVID-19 pandemic has even more significantly impacted college enrollment negatively (National Student Clearinghouse Research Center 2022b). This decade-long decline in enrollment has occurred despite the well-established fact that those with a college degree (any college degree) earn more money than those who do not have a college degree (Dawson et al. 2021a). Chapter 3 of this book discusses population trends related to Millennials and Gen Zs as one reason for this declining trend. Another potential reason for this trend is that the number of public and private non-profit four-year schools has increased since 2009, providing more institutional choices to applicants (US Department of Education 2022).

One bright spot in the decade-long declining trend in college applications is that the decline has been isolated to undergraduate admissions. Graduate programs on the other hand have seen the opposite effect, as enrollment has increased by 10% between 2009 and 2020 (US Department of Education 2022). This period spans a time when both Millennials and Gen Z are entering college. The increase in graduate applications is hopeful news for health professions programs, as these professions require a graduate or professional degree before graduation and licensure. Medical schools, in particular, have experienced about a 16% increase in applicants since 2012, according to the Association of American Medical Colleges (Association of American

Medical Colleges 2021). Inside Higher Ed dubs this the "Fauci Effect," as potential students became increasingly more interested in health professions after living through the COVID-19 worldwide health crises (Burke 2021).

Like medicine, enrollment in colleges of veterinary medicine has increased an average of 2.6% per year from 2011 to 2022 (AACVM 2023). However, there were significant decreases in enrollment in baccalaureate-level nursing programs from 2018 to 2023. Between 2021 and 2022, enrollment in all nursing degree programs decreased except for the Doctor of Nursing Practice degree which increased slightly by 0.6%. The most significant drop was in enrollment for Registered Nurse to Bachelor of Science in Nursing degree programs which decreased by 16.9% (AACN 2023).

Cost of Higher Education

The price associated with attending college is a barrier preventing students from enrolling and staying in college (Kelderman 2021). Students from low- and middle-income families are especially vulnerable to this barrier. Seeking financial aid support is only one mechanism to aid in the cost of college, yet this process can be confusing and cumbersome to families. As discussed in Chapter 3, Gen Z students and their families appreciate value and practicality with spending, thus they are less willing to enter into debt-laden enterprises, like attending college. For these learners, the question of value for price is forefront in the decision to attend college and for how long. Therefore, when it comes to a college education, Gen Zs more than Millennials grapple with the cost and question if the college experience is worth the price tag. In addition, families of Gen Z learners might question if attending college is relevant for a successful career (HelloCampus 2022), which differs from their Millennial predecessors who continue to place significant value on attending college. Further compounding this hesitancy is the question of job availability post-graduation, as well as the need to customize the college experience to fit one's needs. Rather than seeing college as a time to explore personal interests, Gen Z learners prefer the time spent in college to prepare them for a profession (HelloCampus 2022). As a result, Gen Zs prefer majors that prepare them for specific careers. The most popular majors for Gen Zs are the ones with obvious and practical paths, including those in the health professions, computer science, engineering, biology, and sports medicine (HelloCampus 2022). Like Gen Zs, Millennials also covet meaningful careers. However, Millennials are more willing to embrace the cost associated with college tuition because career success is very important to this generation (Seemiller and Grace 2019a).

According to the National Center for Education Statistics, during the 2020 and 2021 academic school years, one of the most common reasons for students enrolled in college to change their plans regarding college attendance was an inability to pay for classes or educational expenses (National Center for Education Statistics 2020a; National Center for Education Statistics 2021). The economic crises spurred by the COVID-19 pandemic was the cause of this trend. Interestingly but not surprisingly, the inability to afford college during this time impacted females more than males. Given declining trends in undergraduate applications, the cost of attending college, and the impact of the COVID-19 pandemic, Forbes magazine asked why bachelor's degrees take four years or more to complete, wondering instead if it was possible to condense the requirements or shorten length to completion (Busteed 2020). This is a relevant question for Gen Z learners as it would result in a less expensive degree path for them and earlier entry into a career, which are two expectations of Generation Z. While innovations around degree completions are being explored across the United States, it is important for health professions to consider the pros and cons of shortening the time to undergraduate degree completion. While this might have benefits for students and their families, especially in short-term cost savings, students will experience the rigors of professional school earlier, and thus might struggle both academically and emotionally. Given the mental health struggles of this student population, earlier entry into a demanding graduate or professional program may also prove difficult to adequately manage.

Recommendations to Increase Enrollment and Manage Cost

While cutting the time to degree completion should be explored for feasibility among institutional stakeholders, other strategies have been proposed to aid students and their families with the cost of college. These include programs negotiating with suppliers for textbook supply packages, ensuring a college degree is worth the time and expense, combating student-centered issues like food insecurity, housing needs, and mental health challenges, and offering tutoring and career advising. As was discussed in previous chapters, unlike Millennials, families of Gen Z students are hyper-focused on the cost of higher education. Therefore, transparency and support around tuition costs are important to reach and retain this generation of students.

While innovative ideas have circulated regarding how undergraduate programs can manage cost, controlling cost is perhaps a more challenging topic within health professions programs, especially those requiring a graduate or professional degree after undergrad. Scholarships have been and continue to be a viable option for many attendees. Yet almost 75% of those with professional doctorates carry student loan debt for attending professional school (Hanson 2022). Among those attending professional school, medical students are the most likely to have student loan debt. Millennials and Gen Zs have taken on the cost of graduate and professional school in hopes of reaping the long-term benefits of a successful career. Gen Zs in particular seek on- and off-campus employment to cover the cost of attending college (Kubaryk 2020a).

In addition, declining undergraduate applications have encouraged colleges to look inward at their recruitment and retention strategies. Organizational missions and practices have been evolving to better align with this changing student body and enrollment numbers. Marketing and communication approaches have intensified, which reaches Millennials and Gen Zs given the amount of time they spend on digital devices. Seeking instant gratification, Gen Zs particularly welcome digital advertising on online platforms, especially when first exploring a program or institution (Seemiller and Grace 2016). Once a student is interested, the more formal campus meeting and tour can follow. This process has evolved in the last few decades, as traditionally, a student's first exposure to campus life was through a physical visit. Gen Zs particularly appreciate communication that is "front and center," so programs should maximize visibility and virtual content around their campus offerings and degree programs (Rhyneer 2021).

Millions of students who start college never finish it, leading to a "completion crisis" (Dawson et al. 2021a, 3). This is, however, not a trend that is unique to Gen Zs. Initiatives, research, and policies have been enacted in the past decade to boost persistence and completion rates for college students. In more recent years, the focus of such initiatives has shifted to newer approaches focused on more comprehensive student services (e.g., case management, mentoring, financial assistance, academic advising, and counseling services) (Dawson et al. 2021a).

There has been implementation in the higher education sphere of initiatives that better support the whole student as they navigate college admission and progression. Such initiatives are timely as Gen Z learners consider college an immersive experience. Traditional college advising focuses on coursework and has largely excluded support on intrapersonal, social, and/or institutional aspects of the college experience. The subsequent paragraphs will highlight innovative institutional practices and structures that have been shown to better support the multi-faceted needs of enrollees. While varying in complexity, delivery, and focus, all the initiatives listed in the following paragraphs take a comprehensive approach to helping students overcome common barriers that can impact progression (Dawson et al. 2021b). These innovations are especially well suited to assist the characteristics of Gen Z and Millennial learners in their college journey and beyond.

- The California State University has identified six operational priorities to define their Graduation Initiative 2025 in an effort to increase degree completion and offer more comprehensive student support (The California State University n.d.). Their six priorities include academic preparation, enrollment management, student engagement and well-being, financial support, data-informed decision making, and administrative barriers. Their distinctive program includes multiple strategies and interventions that engage an assortment of stakeholders.
- Accelerated Study in Associate Programs (ASAP) is another initiative that was originally developed by a university in New York but has expanded to other campuses in the United States. It was designed to provide comprehensive support for up to three years for first-time, full-time, low-income students. Students in the program have access to an adviser who supports the gamut of students' academic, social, and interpersonal needs. Tuition waivers and free books are also offered (Borough of Manhattan Community College, n.d.).
- Inside Track is an independent non-profit provider of coaching services that serves college students across the nation. Coaches support students at the start of college and through the first year, helping them to overcome barriers and plan for success (Inside Track n.d.).
- Monitoring Advising Analytics to Promote Success (MAAPS) was originally launched as a research endeavor at an institution in Georgia to address the lack of institutional "know how" of many low-income, first-generation students. Since inception, it has expanded to multiple states. The program provides students with intensive, proactive advising with targeted interventions (Alamuddin, Rossman, and Kurzweil 2018).
- One Million Degrees is a non-profit organization that offers comprehensive support to community college students in Chicago, Illinois. The program targets low-income students with a grade point average (GPA) of at least 2.0 and pairs students with an adviser whom they meet with on a monthly basis. The adviser works with students to address challenges and create a plan for success. This program offers initiatives (i.e., incentives and scholarships), resources (i.e., workshops), and coaching (One Million Degrees 2022).
- Project QUEST is a non-profit organization that provides comprehensive support to adults seeking degrees to access local, well-paying jobs. The program includes financial support, remedial instruction in certain subjects, counseling, referrals, weekly meetings on life skills, and job placement support (Project QUEST 2021).
- Total Advising Initiative is part of a university's integrated approach to student advising (Tyton Partners and Babson Survey Research Group 2019). The single location aims to provide students with a single

location for provision of academic and professional support. The center increases collaboration between the student and academic affairs.

As with any initiative, cost is a large factor in sustainability. As a result, it is important that student support initiatives target students who will benefit to the largest degree. There is still a lot to learn about the benefits of institutional initiatives.

CHAPTER SUMMARY AND CONCLUSION

Gen Z and Millennial learners have unique characteristics for which college campuses need to be attune. In addition to being individualistic, learners want the campus community to provide them with support outside of the classroom. Initiatives around mental health and well-being are critical to the college experience, and many institutions have taken steps to address gaps in care. Additionally, Gen Zs and Millennials want the guidance and mentorship of advisers, not just for academic support, but also for mental health support and career guidance. As college enrollment fluctuates and tuition increases in the United States, students are seeking guidance and transparency from institutions. While a career in health professions might entice Gen Zs, they are reluctant to acquire significant debt unlike their Millennial counterparts. Some institutions and programs have been innovative, however, and have developed initiatives, structures, and/or programming aimed to meet the needs of Gen Z and Millennials learners. The next chapter extends the conversation on learning and explores Gen Z and Millennial preferences in the classroom setting. Chapter 5 also discusses the factors that educators should consider when designing content and teaching these generations.

Chapter 5

Considerations for Teaching Millennials and Gen Zs in the Classroom

For decades, educators have studied how teaching facilitates learning. While an assortment of pedagogies has been implemented and subsequently published over the years, there is not a one-size-fits all approach that meets the needs of all learners, nor the skill sets of all educators. This is because teaching and learning are both context-bound, meaning that both educators and students—as individuals—matter, and thus contribute to the vibrancy of the learning environment. Individuals must be collectively acknowledged for the context, experiences, and worldviews they carry. This acknowledgment provides opportunities for richer education, departing from the sterility of traditional classroom environments. Acknowledging the uniqueness of Millennial and Gen Z learners and educators, this chapter focuses on considerations for teaching in higher education and the health professions.

Consider this philosophical question: when a new generation of learners is ushered in, is it the role of educators to accommodate learners by updating their teaching practices? Or is it the role of students to conform to the educator's style? This can be visualized by thinking of a seesaw. On one end are educators and on the other end are students. In contemporary education, which side should tilt *more* toward the other in an effort to be accommodating? Or should an equal balance be the desired result? There are an assortment of different answers and beliefs to this question, each having merit. The balance likely lies somewhere in the middle. While educators cannot cater to every student and need, educators do set the stage by modeling certain behaviors and beliefs. To create an inclusive and responsive classroom, educators should lean toward the needs of students by being in tune with their learning preferences and updating teaching approaches in response. It is important to acknowledge that faculty have skill sets around certain teaching methods, and there is a limit to the degree of change that one can comfortably manage. While departing from the safety of one's preferred teaching practice can be uncomfortable, this is where growth occurs. After all, rather than basing pedagogical strategies on existing research, many educators approach teaching using the same discipline-specific models they observed as students (Bowen 2012). This chapter will focus on rationale and strategies for making a contemporary classroom more student centric for Millennials and Gen Zs.

TEACHING AND LEARNING IN FOCUS

It is the educator's responsibility to create a welcoming and inclusive classroom. Students value instructors who are approachable, helpful, and encouraging (Felten and Lambert 2020). This is because these characteristics promote connection and openness. More specifically, for health professions students, the seven teaching qualities valued by pharmacy and nursing students include educators who are approachable/personable, effective communicators, encourages/cares, enthusiastic, knowledgeable, understanding, and have realistic expectations for classroom learning (Groccia et al. 2018). Considering the amount of medical knowledge to learn, it is interesting that health professions students prefer educators who they can relate to over educators who promote critical thinking. Educators can express deep caring for students by offering "relentless welcomes," which are sustained practices of creating a hospitable atmosphere (Felten and Lambert 2020, 20).

Gen Z and Millennial learners view the role of their educators as facilitators rather than preachers. Considering they learn best when provided hands-on experiences, these generations do not like to be lectured to; these students prefer to be involved in the learning process (Prater 2020; Seemiller and Grace 2016). This preference is quite distinct from previous generations. Within health professions, which tends to have very structured curricula, one way to engage students is to offer them options and seek their input where feasible. This allows students to build agency with personal decision making and might include input on elective choices, rotation locations, test dates, and policies around classroom norms. Each generation has preferences for learning modalities and approaches. Luckily for educators who are teaching both Millennials and Gen Z learners, these generations share similarities in their learning and classroom preferences. Both Millennial and Gen Z students want to be stimulated in the classroom *and* included in the learning process. The need for stimulation could be due to their use of digital technology and resultant shortened attention spans. In a scoping review of Gen Z students enrolled in healthcare programs, their learning was stimulated when they could visualize and sense things (Shorey et al. 2021). As a result, they prefer classroom activities that promote active learning and experiences that allow them to observe a behavior before practicing it. The need for inclusivity in the learning environment aligns with Millennials and Gen Zs' needs to promote diversity and belonging on campus, as well as their desire to have autonomy. The next four sections focus on key areas significant to Millennial and Gen Zs regarding classroom learning: digital connectiveness, influence of parents, mentorship dynamics, and inclusive teaching.

Digital Connectiveness

Accessing online resources through the myriad of devices at their disposal, Millennial and Gen Z learners are technologically savvy. It is the desire to be digitally connected that characterizes these generations over others. Gen Zs in particular have never known life without cell phones and Wi-Fi; therefore, they desire immediacy of information. Millennials and Gen Z students, having information at their fingertips, are accustomed to technology in the learning environment. Most students of these generations have laptops, tablets, and smart phones readily accessible, and therefore are digitally connected from the moment they enter the classroom (Seemiller and Grace 2016). While accessibility to technology promotes information access, the sheer breadth of information available can also present complications for students and educators as discussed in Chapters 1 and 2.

Gen Z learners are the first "postliterate" generation (Zarra 2017, 64). This means that, due to their digital connectiveness, internet results or cell phone applications do the thinking for them. Millennials, also being a digitally literate generation, place an overemphasis on information access as well. Both generations have access to information all over the world, and thus think and communicate globally (Szymkowiak et al. 2021). On one hand, accessibility to information improves efficiency and removes barriers. On the other hand, access to technology can impair students' abilities to develop critical thinking skills if they never have to analyze or synthesize information. In addition, searching for information online produces thousands of results, which can be distracting when trying to decide what is relevant. As a result of the volume of information readily available on the internet (Zarra 2017), students are unable to filter and prioritize the most important information in order to direct or solidify their learning. If a quick internet search does not yield relevant results, they tend to move on and not consider alternate sources of information (Zarra 2017).

Technology and Learning

Watching tutorials is an important component of how Millennials and Gen Zs supplement classroom learning. YouTube for example is a popular site that students utilize to enhance instruction (Seemiller and Grace 2016). What is important for educators to realize is that students supplement classroom instruction by accessing information found online, meaning classroom resources are not the sole source of information for students. Therefore, faculty should be aware of what students might view online. Educators, particularly of previous generations, may grapple with the notion that it is their responsibility to create a vibrant and interactive learning environment that requires creative approaches to incorporating technology. Despite this, quick web searches of course material should be conducted to ensure there are no significant discrepancies between what is presented in class and what the students find online. Searching information online ahead of teaching also allows educators to stay up to date with information that students might be accessing. As a result, educators can encourage or discourage the use of certain resources that students might review. It is also important for educators to keep in mind that infusing virtual resources should be for the promotion of student engagement or to enhance learning, and not just for the sake of adding technology that might not be practical or effective.

Of all the generations, Gen Zs have the strongest presence across social media platforms (Szymkowiak et al. 2021). A study on internet use for instructional purposes found that, despite the rapid development of the internet in the 21st century, web-based instruction (defined as using the web as the medium for instruction) played a minor role in contemporary medical education (Vogelsang et al. 2018). Internet-based media were utilized in the classroom by only 28% of teachers in the study. The educators who incorporated web-based instruction however stated that it improved the diversity of the courses and promoted a higher level of student satisfaction. Results of this study demonstrate that while the value of web-based instruction has been established, its implementation is lacking in health professions education.

Interestingly, there is a common misconception that, due to their need to be digitally connected, Gen Zs desire online learning over face-to-face instruction. Rather, it is Millennials and Gen Xers who prefer online instruction over Generation Z (Seemiller and Grace 2019a). Gen Z students thrive in blended learning environments, where instruction is delivered by a mixture of face-to-face and virtual settings. Gen Z students also thrive when allowed to take a more active and autonomous role in their learning. A flipped classroom model is one ideal format for Gen Zs because it promotes independent and application-based learning. A meta-analysis conducted in health professions students found that a flipped classroom approach, which is when students complete pre-work or group work on their own as homework before attending class, yielded significant learning improvements compared with traditional methods of teaching (Hew and Lo 2018).

Technology and the Brain

Consistent use of technology affects the brain in positive and negative ways. When people are constantly using technology, they spend less time engaging with others. A review from neuroscientists articulated several negative consequences of digital technology on brain health (Small et al. 2020). Negative aspects of digital technology included reduced attention spans, impaired emotional and social intelligence, technology addiction, social isolation, impaired cognitive and brain development (particularly in children), and sleep disruptions. Despite this, there are positive aspects of repeated use of digital technology, which include brain stimulation, cognition, multi-tasking, and memory (Small et al. 2020). Repeated reading of digital information activates different brain centers over traditional readings. Through brain imaging, researchers discovered that text reading activates the brain regions that control language, reading, memory, and visualization, whereas repeated digital reading activates the brain in the regions that control decision making, complex reasoning, and vision. This suggests that repeated use of digital searching might be a form of positive brain exercise.

Parental Influence

Both Millennial and Gen Z learners value involvement of parents; however, there are generational differences to note. Millennials prefer to choose the authority figures with which to work, whereas Gen Zs prefer to collaborate with authority (Mohr and Mohr 2017). Millennials were raised by parents who hovered over their development and influenced their decisions (sometimes called helicopter parents). This influenced Millennials' goal-oriented tendencies and placed considerable pressure on them to achieve (Swanzen 2018). According to Seemiller and Grace, for Millennials, "being a parent of a college student has become an identity all to itself" (2016, 194). While parents of Gen Zs influence them, the parental relationship is different from Millennials; it is reminiscent of a trusted mentor relationship or co-pilot instead of an enforcer or influencer (Seemiller and Grace 2016). More than half of Gen Zs consult their parents on matters important to them, and beyond that, consider their parents as their ultimate role model more so than Millennials do (Seemiller and Grace 2016). Parents of Generation Z are typically from the Gen X era and therefore favor pragmatism. As a result, these parents encourage development of independence resulting in a generation that values parental involvement as equally as Millennials but perhaps feels more empowered by the dynamic (Mohr and Mohr 2017; Seemiller and Grace 2016).

Unlike some of the other areas discussed in this chapter, parental involvement is an area where Millennials and Gen Zs diverge. It is an important distinction for educators, as the differences have implications in the classroom. For Millennials, heavy parental involvement creates ambition and thus the achievement of educational goals. However, it has led to entitlement, self-interest, and lack of decision-making abilities among this group (Mohr and Mohr 2017). Millennials may lack the ability to set the course for themselves while feeling a sense of over-confidence in their ability to do so. Educators will thus need to ensure Millennials can grow their personal agency and decision-making abilities, despite it being uncomfortable for them. On the other hand, parents of Gen Zs have shaped them in more collaborative and supportive ways than parents of Millennials. This has led to a generation that is open minded and interactive, yet less focused and less creative (Mohr and Mohr 2017). Gen Zs will therefore seek collaboration in the learning environment with the expectation that all viewpoints are considered. Educators will need to ensure the student voice is heard. Inclusive teaching is explored in a subsequent section.

Mentorship Dynamics

Teachers represent other authority figures that influence Millennials and Gen Z learners. Within this relationship, both Millennials and Gen Zs are more apt to dissolve the more traditional hierarchical structures characteristic of Gen X and Boomers, in favor of heightened collaboration. As discussed in Chapters 1 and 2, newer generations are more diverse than prior generations. Therefore, in an effort to confront injustices and achieve greater appreciation of differences, Millennials and Gen Zs might question the positionality and beliefs of their mentors. Being questioned can be uncomfortable, especially those in a position of power like teachers in a classroom. Interestingly, the more powerful the person, the greater tendency there is to assume that their rules are the norm. Lammert and Malek Ash (2022) state that power manifests in unwritten rules. As an educator, becoming more aware of the unwritten rules in classrooms and institutions is a crucial step in understanding the power dynamics that influence the student-instructor relationship. In reference to the sentiment discussed at the beginning of this chapter, acknowledging differences among students is a significant *and* powerful first step in contemporary teaching, and should be a minimum expectation of all educators.

In health professions education, students typically matriculate through programs as a cohort. Since students tend to progress at the same pace, there is less personalization in the curricula with regard to which class to take and when. This can create a sense of homogenization for students and perpetuates the notion that students' identities as individuals are not relevant. However, this is untrue as development of both personal and professional identities contribute to learning (Cruess et al. 2015). Homogenized progression could be perceived by students as "the normal" approach to their schooling experiences, meaning students might internalize this as their personal identities do not matter. Educators instinctively know that this is not the case, so perpetuating this standard is likely unintentional or subconscious. Therefore, an important question for educators to consider is this: in the face of the standardized curricula that is characteristic of health professions education, how can students feel that they are important and accepted as individuals? There are myriad ways to answer this question, and educators should explore answers within their contexts. Despite there not being a holistic picture of what mentorship looks like in health professions education literature, this chapter proposes that educators consider how their relationships with students should focus on relationship building. As Lammert and Malek Ash (2022) state, mentoring relationships should be more reflective and less evaluative.

Millennials and Gen Zs seek feedback from mentors, so the provision of feedback is valued regardless of generation. However, *how* the feedback is given is what is important for these generations. When providing feedback with a traditional mindset, mentors often take an unintentional power-laden approach, which is evaluative in nature. This means that the mentor renders judgment on whether the mentee's work is acceptable or not. Not only does this create intellectual dependence on behalf of learners, but it perpetuates the power dynamics and the "not good enough" mentality of learners (Lammert and Malek Ash 2022). In health professions curricula, this approach is unavoidable though, at least to a degree. Training to become a professional requires standardized evaluation practices and feedback from an expert. However, there are areas in health professions education where reflective feedback can replace evaluative feedback. Mentoring relationships focused on reflection utilize co-constructive dialogue, targeted questioning, and data to facilitate discussions that encourage students to reach their own conclusions. This approach is more future focused and lessens the hierarchy in the student-educator relationship. An example of this is students interacting with patients. As a mentor, instead of critiquing/evaluating how the student interacted with the patient, which is difficult to standardize anyway, ask the student to reflect on how they thought it went as a first step. Then, consider how your observations (i.e., data) as a mentor can *support* the student in deriving meaning from the patient interaction.

Millennials and Gen Zs expect accessibility from faculty. This might create dissonance when expectations of learners do not match realities of how educators manage their time. Waljee, Chopra, and Saint (2020) propose three areas of consideration that educators should keep in mind when managing the mentorship dynamic with students.

1. Scheduled versus As Needed Engagement—The propensity for instant communication among Gen Z and Millennials necessitates their need for rapid turnaround and quick responses. Educators and mentors are balancing multiple demands that students often cannot appreciate. They might also be less connected to digital communication than their students, and therefore often have less on-the-fly availability.
2. Flat versus Pyramidal Infrastructure—Millennials and Gen Zs appreciate collaboration, groupthink, broad access, and transparency in decision making, and cognitive diversity more readily than older generations. This is a flatter, or more equalized paradigm. This approach might be in contrast to educators of prior generations who are more accustomed to hierarchical or pyramidal communication and decision making, which is when decisions are made "from above."
3. Purpose versus Process—Purpose dictates decisions for both Millennials and Gen Zs. While Millennials tend to be more idealistic and Gen Zs more pragmatic, purpose is still central to decision making for both generations. As a result, measuring success might look different for the newer generations as it is more aligned with an individual's purpose, more so than societal expectations.

These three considerations point to the need for a greater understanding of the differences between Millennial and Gen Z students and the generational cohorts who educate them. This is accomplished through heightened communication and expression of expectations, which largely falls on faculty to initiate and sustain. Communication becomes more fluid and expected once relationships are established. Hence, the messaging in this chapter is largely focused on the importance of cultivating relationships with students (more information will be presented in the "Inclusive Teaching" section).

Mentorship keeps students as the center point. While it might be difficult for educators to forgo some of their working day in favor of student development, it is a necessary component. Expecting students to be independently responsible for their educational experiences is an antiquated mindset that perpetuates existing social inequities and overlooks the important role that educators and institutions play in student success. This is where mentorship plays a central role: being a co-pilot in the student experience. Mentors are not alone in this, as students too must also engage in the dynamic. Expectations of students include developing relationships, asking questions, and exploring curiosities (Felten and Lambert 2020). Characteristics of meaningful mentoring conversations include (1) creating space for students to be heard and seen as human; (2) the provision of "nitty-gritty" guidance and knowledge; (3) "warm handoffs" to other resources that facilitate yet more relationships; (4) planning conversations during low or transitional periods in students' lives; and (5) leaving legacies that endure beyond the dialogue (Felten and Lambert 2020, 136).

Mentorship Conversations

Authors of *Relationship-Rich Education* state that relationships are the "heartbeat" of institutions (Felten and Lambert, 2020, 1). After conducting hundreds of interviews with educators, administrators, and students across a variety of US institutions, the authors derived four intersecting principles to guide education that is relationship-rich: (1) ensure every student feels valued by genuinely welcoming them to campus and expressing deep care; (2) inspire students to learn by showcasing passion for the topic and inspiring curiosity; (3) encourage students to develop a network of significant relationships with peers and faculty (beyond the formal structures of advising); and (4) encourage students to explore questions around meaning and purpose.

College is a natural time for students to ask questions about themselves and the world. While questions are natural, navigating these conversations to promote meaning-making requires authentic dialogue and guidance from mentors. One such question to facilitate discussion was proposed in the work by Felten and Lambert: "Who are you becoming for other people, not just yourself?" (2020, 36). Mentorship is not (necessarily) about formal conversations and scheduled meetings; in fact, authentic mentorship is often created in informal spaces or serendipitous meetings. Table 5.1 provides mentorship opportunities for educators which enhance relationships with students to overcome the dissonance in generational world views.

While it is important for educators to keep mentorship central to their role, it can often be challenging to embrace mentorship, particularly for those who educate students within health professions education. There are multiple reasons for this. First, health professions cohorts are often large in size, which creates barriers for educators who seek to build individual relationships and mentor students. It is almost impossible to personally connect with all students in this environment. Second, mentors may also feel less prepared to help students navigate their educational experiences or assist in the development of student identity due to the fact that faculty trained in science, technology, engineering, and mathematics (STEM) and/or clinical practice, like those in health professions education, are not necessarily trained in nor geared toward mentorship. Third, institutions do not typically place value nor offer incentives for time spent mentoring students. As a result, these factors might

Table 5.1 Ways to Cultivate Relationships with Students

Relationship-Building Approach	*Definition*
Micromentoring	Micromentoring is a more efficient approach to traditional mentorship. It entails more frequent and rapid meetings with the goal of providing feedback on narrow topics. It might entail a quick check-in or asking a pointed question.
Reverse Mentoring	In a flattened structure, reverse mentoring allows and encourages students to provide feedback and perspective to older generations rather than the reverse. This can empower learners and promote efficiency in collaboration.
Mentorship Teams	This is a teams-approach to mentorship, rather than an individualized approach. It requires collaboration. This strategy leverages the strengths of mentors to capitalize on the overall influence of mentorship.
Peer Mentoring	Not all mentoring has to be done by the educator. Connecting with immediate others (i.e., peers) is a meaningful strategy for student connection. Students may be more vulnerable with peers over mentors.
Making Relationships a Cultural Priority	Creating a culture that prioritizes relationships is a collective and sustained responsibility. This is the idea of intentionally fostering a culture that allows relationships to flourish. Even one faculty who embraces a mentorship mentality can help the idea take root and spread among others.
Mentoring Mindset	This is a shift from the *act* of mentoring a student to the *internalization* of mentorship as a component of identity. This is an intentional process that requires an evolution in mindset.
Informal Conversations	Informal conversations with students are undervalued and underutilized. Get-to-know-you questions are a meaningful first step in students feeling seen and building a mentoring relationship.
Developing as a Mentor	Developing others starts with oneself. Educators would benefit from reflecting on questions related to their capacity to mentor, including: 1. Am I using my time to meaningfully engage with others? 2. Am I listening to what I am hearing and trying to understand (rather than respond)? 3. Am I offering practical advice, encouragement, and support? 4. Am I connecting students with other valuable resources who might also mentor them? 5. Am I helping to create spaces and structures that ensure mentorship is promoted? 6. What am I learning about myself through mentorship?

Source: Adapted from Waljee, Chopra, and Saint (2020), and Felten and Lambert (2020)

impede educators' abilities to meaningfully mentor students. A more in-depth exploration of the role of mentoring in the classroom and in the clinical environment will be explored in Chapter 9.

Inclusive Teaching

Being socially conscious, Gen Z and Millennial students appreciate an inclusive and diverse learning environment more so than prior generations. This was influenced by their exposure to a wide range of different people (Seemiller and Grace 2016). In fact, safety, well-being, and inclusion are as important as academic rigor for Gen Z learners (Selingo 2021). In addition, Gen Zs believe colleges and universities need to be doing more to support these initiatives, including creating a more inclusive and safer environment—in essence, a community. Inclusion in classrooms is prompted by dialogue, which in turn "gives life" to the student voice. Inclusivity is more than fitting in; it is about belonging and thus feeling accepted as a person. Establishing connections with others is important because it makes an individual feel accepted. However, making connections with others is only one facet of cultivating inclusiveness. With generations growing more diverse, educators must consider how the social environment of the classroom creates a sense of belonging, equity, and inclusion.

Over the last few decades, research indicates that underrepresented students have been departing from STEM education due to reduced feelings of social belonging in these fields (Dewsbury and Brame 2019). As educators, being inclusive requires being intentional about recognizing others and mitigating biases. This is specifically important for STEM educators. Inclusion is built on the quality of social relationships; students need to know educators care about their success as individuals. STEM faculty are formally trained as scientists and not educators. As such, scientists are trained to gather, analyze, and report data objectively, which is valuable in research contexts but might be limiting in the classroom. As a result, scientist-educators might be inclined to approach their teaching with the world view that objectivity is important, and subjectivity is a form of bias. Doing so would minimize their presence in the classroom and the uniqueness they bring to the learning environment.

Lecturing is a prevalent form of material delivery in health professions, which focuses on the trained expert delivering information to the trainee. This approach is hierarchical as educators are at "the top" as the experts. In addition, it suppresses the instructor's identity in favor of unidirectional teaching (Dewsbury and Brame 2019), while also removing social connectiveness from the classroom. Given the learning preferences of Millennial and Gen Z health professions students, an active learning format where information is delivered in short bursts, rather than hour-long lectures is most effective for these generations (Prater 2020). Not only does this stimulate learning but it creates a rich and inclusive classroom that fosters social development. Outside of active learning approaches (which are student centered), other ways to foster inclusivity in the learning environment include developing self-awareness as an educator, embracing empathy, fostering a positive and supportive classroom environment, making student-centered instructional choices that promote the student voice, and creating synergy between the learning environment and institutional support structures (Dewsbury and Brame 2019).

The simple practice of incorporating more student-centered teaching approaches is one step toward a more inclusive environment. In many cases, this might be active learning pedagogies, like team-based learning, problem-based learning, and flipped classroom. Dewsbury (2017) states that it is not the degree of active learning that creates inclusivity; rather it is the degree of the instructor-student dialogue that matters. He also states that inclusive pedagogy includes active learning, but active learning is not necessarily inclusive. This can mean that certain pedagogical choices are appropriate for some contexts but not all (Dewsbury and Brame 2019). Implementation of active learning should focus beyond the strategy itself and consider the broader social contexts that influence the nature of their implementation (Dewsbury 2017). This requires unpacking the lived experiences of underrepresented or marginalized students and taking steps to mitigate the negative aspects of those experiences. For health professions educators, attention should also be given to diversity in patient cases, panels, and assessments. Additionally, further training and development in cultural competency and equitable classroom practices would benefit educators in the promotion of inclusive teaching.

Inclusivity is critical for Gen Zs and Millennials classroom experiences. Pedagogy, which embraces inclusiveness and places value on students' voices, starts with questioning ourselves as educators. After all, educators cannot simply detach themselves from content delivery and teaching. "Central to inclusiveness is an understanding of self (the instructor) and student" (Dewsbury 2017, 4). Identity development helps educators to understand themselves *and* their students better, thus creating space to cultivate authentic relationships that support students' needs. Even with this value in mind, promoting inclusive practices might be uncomfortable for educators. It requires taking a step out of one's comfort zone in order to develop personal and professional identities, dialogue and interact with students, implement active learning pedagogies, and sustain mindfulness over the long-term.

Transitioning Away from "Office of Disability Services"

Recognizing students with disabilities as individuals capable of thriving in the learning environment is a component of inclusive teaching. Research indicates that labeling someone as "disabled" can have negative effects on identity (Akin and Huang 2019). This makes practical sense as placing labels on people, any labels, can lead to stereotypes and stigma. Gen Z students with their inclination toward social justice and equality are sensitive to stereotyping. The National Center for Education Statistics reported that in 2015–2016 almost 20% of undergraduate students who attended college had a disability (2018). In medical education, Meeks et al. (2021) reported a discrepancy in the number of students who had anonymously reported having a disability and the number of students who were willing to disclose their disability to receive accommodations. Further, 35% of programs had disability disclosure procedures in place that did not align with Association with American Medical Colleges (AAMC) recommendations.

Students with disabilities are those living with one or more of the following conditions, either visible and non-visible: blindness or visual impairment (which cannot be corrected by wearing glasses), hearing impairment (e.g., deaf or hard of hearing), orthopedic or mobility impairment, speech or language impairment, learning, mental, emotional, or psychiatric condition, or other health impairment or problem. In recent years, many institutions have transitioned the designation of their disability services office in favor of a more inclusive title such as the Office of Accessibility. An office with "disability" in the title has a negative connotation and highlights the limitations of having a disability; whereas labeling an office with "accessibility" in the title has a more positive connotation and reframes the focus from what students cannot do to what students can do.

Teamwork versus Individual Work

Consideration of student preferences around teamwork versus individual work is another component of inclusive teaching. Millennials enjoy teamwork and view it as an expected part of the educational experience (Howe and Strauss 2003). This is due to their need to create a sense of community on campus and their orientation toward civic engagement. Uniquely though, Millennials can divide up tasks using text or video messaging without feeling the need to physically meet (Seemiller and Grace 2016). Gen Zs on the other hand prefer to work independently even if physically together, collaborating only when it enhances learning and is on their terms (Seemiller and Grace 2016). An example of this is the utility of collaborative spaces (e.g.,

Google Docs) that allow for collaboration without the interactive teamwork component. Individual work is preferred by Gen Zs because they can control the pace and environment with which learning occurs (Seemiller and Grace 2019a). Despite the preference for independent work, this does not mean Gen Zs like to be isolated from their social environment. As mentioned in a previous section, they crave connections with others, specifically in a digital format.

For educators creating high impact teamwork for Millennials and Gen Zs, consider how projects can promote individual learning *before* collaboration is required. Traditionally, educators may assign a project requiring teamwork, then collect the final product at the deadline. This approach may not align with Millennial and Gen Z preferences. Luckily, with a few tweaks, it can become more meaningful for these generations of learners. There are two practical ways to enhance teamwork in this regard: (1) having students work on the same section independently, coming together to synthesize *after* the section has been drafted by all members; and (2) taking into consideration the strengths of all team members, then equitably assigning out roles that promote these strengths (Seemiller and Grace 2019a). Utilizing these two strategies for effective teamwork promotes learning because students are better prepared to engage with others. It also makes teamwork more efficient, which reduces the perception that teamwork is busywork.

Educators must also consider the social implications of teamwork preferences. Considering the diverse demographics of students in these generations, it might be difficult for some students to find their niche or establish their social identity on campus (Howe and Strauss 2003). The consequence of which is feeling isolated. Much research has confirmed that creating a sense of belonging is a crucial piece in maximizing learning and development. Therefore, while students may push back with assignments that require teamwork, it can be a worthy struggle for learners. Educators should be cautioned against removing all teamwork just because students may not prefer it. When considering teamwork, the goals for educators should be to create opportunities that promote learning, social connectiveness, and collaboration to mitigate isolation and promote belonging and inclusion. Additional attention is given to the role of teamwork in Chapter 8 when exploring team dynamics in the context of interprofessional education.

CHAPTER SUMMARY AND CONCLUSION

Educators should remember that teaching is not *just* about content delivery but includes the people involved (Zarra 2017). Millennials and Gen Z learners thrive in learning environments that promote relationships and inclusivity.

Educators should ensure they are building rapport with students yet also encouraging students to build relationships with peers. Mentorship is an important factor for Millennials and Gen Zs in the college experience as they have a strong foundation of family support.

It is the role of the educator to encourage students to explore curiosities within an inclusive classroom environment. The incorporation of technology can assist instruction but should only be integrated strategically to enhance teaching or learning. There are several considerations for health professions educators to promote a student-centric classroom. Chapter 6 continues the discussion of learning with a focus on clinical and lab skill development within health professions education. The emphasis of the next chapter centers on competency-based education and immersive technologies within the context of skill development.

Chapter 6

Assessing Competency-Based Education and Navigating Clinical/Lab Skills with Millennial and Generation Z Learners

The competitive and globalized economy has lead employers and professional organizations to expect higher education institutions to produce graduates with the relevant skills and competencies for practice (Sistermans 2020). Preparing learners for entry into practice requires health professions educators to identify key and strategic educational experiences that mimic the healthcare environment. As Miller noted, "To fulfill that broader objective, graduates must also know how to use the knowledge they have accumulated, for otherwise they may be little more than 'idiot savants'" (1990, S63). To ensure that learners are prepared to navigate the clinical environment, the incorporation of competency-based education (CBE) supplemented with hands-on, real-world simulation experiences offered through clinical and skills lab activities are essential to ensure that students are prepared for the realities of practice. Furthermore, this curricular realignment has led health professions education programs to also integrate case-based and/or problem-based learning into their curriculum to compliment the competency-based framework being implemented to meet marketplace demands. This chapter will explore the history of CBE, CBE adoption within health professions education, the role of clinical skills development as well as other CBE identified assessment best practices. It will also examine how multigenerational learners influence the development of these experiences to gain a better understanding of how to develop, implement, and manage the learning environment for these student populations.

COMPETENCY-BASED EDUCATION FOR CLINICAL COMPETENCE

The role of CBE within health professions education has expanded over the last decade as educators and accrediting bodies push for outcomes-driven student learning rather than process-driven outcomes (Desy, Reed, and Wolanskyj 2017). Yet, an ongoing challenge has been the lack of a consistent definition for CBE as well as an agreed upon approach to observe and assess it (Hodges et al. 2019). For the purposes of this text, the authors agree with Hodges et al.'s definition, "Competency-based education is an outcomes-based approach that focuses not on teaching, but the design, implementation, assessment, and evaluation of an educational program" (2019, 675). However, the authors will examine other discipline-specific definitions of CBE later in this chapter.

This need for outcomes-driven learning aligns with the evolving expectations of the healthcare system. Healthcare systems thrive on patient-centered and quality-focused outcomes and the next generation of healthcare providers must be prepared to take on this charge upon entry into practice. To ensure that learners are prepared for these expectations, educators are first charged with establishing the critical thinking and problem-solving skills required to produce lifelong learners. However, before those areas are explored, this chapter will first delve into how learners will be evaluated for these competency-driven skills by exploring the role of competency-based education.

Competency-Based Education Defined

Competency-based education carries significant esteem in higher education, as it facilitates career readiness in a student-centered manner (Frank 2010). CBE serves as a framework for educators as it intends to prepare students to be able to demonstrate the knowledge, skills, and attitudes affiliated with the intended competency prior to completing their academic program (Hodges et al. 2019). Schools are turning to CBE for a variety of reasons, one of which is because it serves as a means to increase access for non-traditional learners (Lurie and Garrett 2017) and allows students to progress at their own pace. CBE is also thought to improve completion rates, align instruction with workforce needs, broaden innovation, clarify expected learning outcomes, and lower tuition costs. With these benefits in mind, the competency-based framework is an ideal curricular structure for college and university programs to consider.

CBE was born decades ago out of a need to reframe curricular processes away from pathways and procedures. The need for employees *to be able to do* rather than *to know* became critical, especially in industrialized countries (Frank et al. 2010). Competency-based education was therefore conceptualized, reorienting education's focus from instruction to outcomes, staking its claim that *all* students will learn something that is measurable (Killen 2000). Because of the workforce focus, CBE serves as an insurance proxy for employers, confirming a graduate's performance is closely linked to the criteria of his or her specialty (Harris et al. 2010). With this in mind, external stakeholders may participate in the competency-development process (Gervais 2016).

CBE gained popularity as an educational framework in medical education in the early 1900s (Sistermans 2020) and in more recent times, this curricular framework has begun to branch out to other health professions education programs. The Education Policy and Accreditation Standards proposed in 2008 by the Council of Social Work Education stressed the value of CBE and presented professional competencies for the first time (McGuire and Lay, 2020). In 2019, the American Association of Colleges of Nursing published an updated version of *Essentials*, which has served as a curricular guide since the 1980s (Lewis, Rebeschi, and Hunt 2022). This guide articulated the need for competency-based education within all levels of nursing programs (American Association of Colleges of Nursing [AACN] 2021). Pharmacy education is still assessing the role of competency-based education within its curricular framework with the American Association of Colleges of Pharmacy (AACP) establishing a joint task force in July 2021 to evaluate the advantages and disadvantages of this curricular approach and to assess if the pharmacy education curriculum allows for the flexibility required to integrate CBE into its educational offerings (AACP Competency-Based Education Task Force 2022).

There have been various attempts to operationalize the definition of CBE in the extant literature. Still, there is no common definition for competency-based education. Within the context of higher education, two recent definitions display the most prominence. Both are captured here, attesting to the explanatory challenge of such a dynamic process. The first definition, purported from medical literature, asserts that CBE is "an approach to preparing [learners] for practice that is fundamentally oriented to graduate outcome abilities and organized around competencies derived from an analysis of societal and patient needs. It de-emphasizes time-based training and promises greater accountability, flexibility, and learner-centeredness" (Frank et al. 2010, 636). A second definition, expressed in educational literature, states "an outcome-based approach to education incorporates modes of instructional delivery and assessment efforts designed to evaluate mastery of learning by students through their demonstration of the knowledge, attitudes, values, skills, and behaviors required for the degree sought" (Gervais 2016, 99). Both definitions, structurally different, yet conditionally similar, carry equal relevance and merit. In the subsequent paragraphs, an exploration of how different health professions disciplines define competency-based education will be provided.

CBE as Defined in Social Work Education

The adoption of the 2008 Education Policy and Accreditation Standards (EPAS) marked the acceptance of competency-based education as the curricular framework for this health professions discipline (McGuire and Lay 2020). Social Work defines CBE in two manners. They articulate what CBE is from a curricular approach, "an outcomes-oriented approach to curriculum design," and what it means for social work competence, "the ability to integrate and apply social work knowledge, values, and skills to practice situations in a purposeful, intentional and professional manner to promote human and community well-being" (Council of Social Work Education [CSWE] 2015, 6). Over time, the definition of social work competence has shifted slightly with the 2022 EPAS defining it as "the ability to integrate and apply social work knowledge, values, skills, and cognitive and affective processes to practice situations in a culturally responsive, purposeful, intentional, and professional manner to promote human and community well-being" (CSWE 2022, 7).

CBE as Defined in Nursing Education

The publication of five core competencies by the Institute of Medicine (IOM 2003) served as the impetus for nursing education to explore competency-based education as a curricular framework. However, it took almost 20 years for the American Association of Colleges of Nursing (AACN) to craft their own competency-based framework to support nursing education best practices and to establish their discipline-specific definition of CBE. The AACN defines competency-based education as "a system of instruction, assessment, feedback, self-reflection, and academic reporting that is based on students demonstrating that they have learned the knowledge, attitudes, motivations, self-perceptions, and skills expected of them as they progress through their education" (2021, 1).

CBE as Defined in Pharmacy Education

Pharmacy education as a whole is still in its infancy regarding CBE, with limited evidence within the literature of the profession's adoption of CBE as a discipline (Katoue and Schwinghammer. 2020). However, the profession is beginning to examine competency-based education and its place within its curricular framework. The work of the AACP CBE Task Force proposed the following definition for competency-based pharmacy education (CBPE), "an outcomes-based curricular model of an organized framework of competencies (knowledge, skills, attitudes) for pharmacists to meet healthcare and societal needs" (2022, 18). Lastly, they identified five essential elements: (1) meets healthcare and societal needs, (2) outcomes-based, (3) de-emphasizes time, (4) creates a learner-centered culture, and (5) includes authentic strategies for teaching and learning that aligns to assessments (AACP CBE Task Force 2022).

CBE Elements

The central tenets of competency-based education are that learning has a purpose and that knowledge builds in a cumulative manner. The purpose(s) of learning are expressed in unambiguous learning expectations, called outcomes or competencies. The three elements, knowledge, skills, and abilities are present within a competency, and the mastery of these three elements within the performance of a role or job demonstrates the fulfillment of this competency (Hodges et al. 2019). The outcomes are focused on developing "the whole" learner (Gervais 2016). Therefore, CBE benefits students by endorsing career readiness and fostering holistic personal development.

The competency-based educational framework consists of four critical features: (1) focuses on outcomes; (2) places emphasis on abilities; (3) reduces emphasis on time-based training; and (4) promotes learner-centeredness (Gruppen et al. 2016; Hodges et al. 2019). Progression is demonstrated through a systematic process: knowledge acquisition to skills development to knowledge application (Hodges et al. 2019). However, the CBE design process is neither simple nor linear. Rather, its framework ensures the inextricable and logical linkage between academic planning and student learning (Killen 2000). The core curricular dimensions, outcomes, teaching, and assessments are strategically and intentionally developed in a "designing back" fashion (Killen 2000, 3). Using this backward approach, broad learning expectations, called competencies or outcomes, are crafted, and agreed upon by stakeholders (Gervais 2016; Harris et al. 2010). Seeing as though the initial competencies are expansive and comprehensive, they represent assessment and instructional challenges. Breaking these broad statements down and stratifying them into component parts makes it easier to align them with assessments and instruction. The breaking-down process is somewhat flexible and context-specific; it continues until the outcomes are measurable or until they are course-level appropriate. It is important to note how scholars differentiate the terms competencies, goals, and objectives. Competencies, which emphasize outcomes or a "realized ability," are written in the present tense and based on what learners should know or be able to demonstrate at the end of their education (Gervais 2016, 100). Conversely, goals are focused on the future and do not carry criteria to measure their attainment. Objectives, on the other hand, are more teacher-centric, focused on what the instructor must contrive in order to produce an overt student behavior. All three terms have varying utility in CBE models.

Breaking down a competency into its various components also benefits learners. Competencies should be regarded as "ingredients of competence" (Frank et al. 2010, 641). As a result, these "pieces" allow designers to visualize the content in multiple ways, encouraging them to intentionally expose students to information at various intervals and intensities. The idea of deliberate exposure can also be expressed in terms of vertical and horizontal understanding: students master sections of the content within a course or unit (vertical understanding) while also integrating their learning across the entire curriculum (horizontal understanding) (Gervais 2016). Designing curriculum with content repetition encourages instructors to view learning with appropriate expectations of mastery in mind. It also alleviates the overwhelming desire some feel to deliver all relevant content at once. Within CBE, instructors still maintain high expectations of their learners, yet their teaching approaches are recalibrated with the understanding that successful learning reinforces further learning (Killen 2000).

Key principles of CBE are explained by Frank et al. (2010). First, curricula must focus on outcomes, and outcomes must emphasize abilities. To align with CBE's purpose that education is for holistic development, instructors must expand their understanding of student learning beyond cognition (or "knowing") as the only value or necessity for building competence. Students acquiring knowledge through instructor bestowment is an antiquated approach and is generally not encouraged in CBE practices. Holistic, learner-centered outcomes therefore emphasize the procurement of additional capacities to cognition, like abilities, skills, and attitudes. These outcomes also stem from industry expectations, therefore ensuring that meeting the learning goals prepares students for their careers. It is important to note that while skills and competencies share some commonalities, their functions are different. Specifically, "skills encompass 'what' activities are needed for a task or job behavior," whereas "competency is 'how' a skill is to be translated into a performance of a job-required behavior" (Hodges et al. 2019, 676).

Another CBE principle mandates that curricula should de-emphasize time-based training (Frank et al. 2010). This means that engagement in a particular educational experience should not be limited to a defined time-frame. Rather, the CBE model suggests that students move through content at varying rates. Killen explains the influence of time on learning, articulating that time should be viewed as a "flexible resource rather than the principal factor that controls access to learning" (2000, 8). Relinquishing arbitrary time-bound restrictions on learning allows teachers to shift their focus from *when* something was learned, to *what* was actually gained, encouraging authentic progression and individualized matriculation. CBE asserts that students should have ongoing opportunities to learn the information, which reinforces another CBE principle that assessments should determine how well information was learned, rather than the degree to which it was retained at a particular time.

The last principle promotes learner engagement, emphasizing that students should be the unequivocal centerpieces of every learning experience (Frank et al. 2010). This practice moves instructors away from singularly focusing on their teaching to acknowledging the uniqueness of students (Killen 2000). Centering students requires instructors to relinquish control of their desire to filter or structure what students are learning and how they are learning it in favor of less direct teaching approaches. The recommendations for how to teach within a competency-based framework are loose and ill-defined. Rather, what is important is the overarching goal of a learner-centered classroom: for learning to be reasonable and desirable for students in a way that promotes their self-confidence and challenges them by new means. Learner-centeredness can be exemplified by a variety of teaching methods; examples include purposeful dialogue around the learning outcomes, expanding opportunities for practical hands-on experiences, and ensuring students strive to reach difficult goals (Killen 2000). In each example, teaching focus is shifted away from teachers, whose role should be less direct and more supportive.

CBE Assessments

Competency-based assessments are directly mapped to the desired outcomes, and therefore serve as mechanisms to evaluate *individual* student performance and facilitate authentic evaluation of individualized learning (Harris et al. 2010). Competencies must also be measurable and observable (Hodges et al. 2019). Although competency-based assessments may flex as learners progress, scholars still consider them as valid tools for measuring learning because they "move us closer to the actual performance of a clinician" (Harris et al. 2010, 647). The authenticity of competency-based assessments should embolden learners to shift their ideas of success away from venerating final grades in favor of acknowledging their overall comprehension. The benefit to this shift is multi-factorial; it reduces reliance on arbitrary grade thresholds (e.g., 75%), removes attendance and participation as indicators of success (Bral and Cunningham 2016), and reminds educators of the importance of learner-centeredness.

Although little consensus exists on how to develop competency-based assessments and when to administer them (McIntyre-Hite 2016), two areas remain clear: the starting point for crafting assessments should always be the outcomes and assessments should always contribute to the nexus of student learning. Killen articulates this sentiment nicely, stating that "learning is a process of continually restructuring prior knowledge, not just adding to it" (2000, 18). Therefore, assessments should help students connect new information to their prior understanding in a meaningful way. Because of this, CBE assessments are not meant to "weed-out" students. Rather, the goal is to provide them with multiple opportunities to learn the concept or to demonstrate their competence. This encourages the design of assessments to promote equity, as assessments should only cover information students have had the opportunity to learn (Cleary and Breathnach 2017; Killen 2000). The complexity and multidimensional nature of student learning can create challenges when assessing a student's progression within identified performance areas; however, student progression typically occurs in a linear fashion (Hodges et al. 2019).

Student-centered assessments, a hallmark of CBE, encourage the use of criterion-oriented evaluations, rather than norm-referenced testing (Frank et al. 2010; Harris et al. 2010; Iobst et al. 2010). This means that judging a student's learning should be based on a continuous comparison to themselves and not "the norm." It also means that the specific elements of a satisfactory performance are determined in advance of the assessment (de Villiers 2006). Therefore, CBE scholars encourage the use of both formative and summative assessment strategies, as long as they are authentic (i.e., direct and representative) (Bral and Cunningham 2016). Formative assessments should be incorporated within or around instructional time and are designed to foster flexibility, encourage feedback, allow for natural progression, and boost collaboration (Bierer et al. 2008; Iobst et al. 2010; Killen 2000). Their aim is to measure learning *progress* toward the competency or outcome. Therefore, they are highly specific to the contextual factors in a classroom. On the other hand, summative assessments are also important for CBE. Being the pre-identified method of ensuring expectations are met, they are fundamental to assessing student readiness for work in an intended field.

Critiques of CBE

Implicit within competency-based education is the assumption that all learners have the capacity to succeed, as this framework requires students make connections across subjects and carry significant responsibility in their own learning (Killen 2000). Although CBE assists learners in doing difficult things well, can everyone meet the predetermined standard? If unsure, programs may feel that educational standards should be lowered to ensure links are easy for students to make between subject matter. It should be clear, however, that low educational standards encourage mediocre performance, which is contradictory to the values of CBE.

There is also a concern that competency-based education may devalue traditional subject matter or academic freedom. If outcomes are derived from core competencies, and instructors are handed specific competencies or outcomes to teach, they may perceive this as a threat to academic freedom (de Villiers 2006; Killen 2000). Seeing as though CBE interrogates long-held beliefs regarding teaching, buy-in can be a barrier for programs who wish to use it. This was demonstrated in a study conducted by Rainwater (2015), who found that CBE implementation requires devotion of significant time, as well as adoption of new teaching methods.

While competency-based education allows students the latitude to progress at their own pace, this flexibility can also create anxiety within faculty and has the potential to impact a program financially. Traditionally, health professions programs have been lock-step with students progressing through the curriculum at a set pace; the adoption of CBE may be challenging for faculty who have taught in these programs for a number of years who are used to structured progression. Administrators must be prepared to provide the development needed to assist faculty with making the transition to this new curricular framework.

Lastly, seeing as though outcomes are heavily ability-based, instructors may not espouse CBE due to the belief it is too behavioristic (Killen 2000). Others may be fundamentally opposed to the idea of having to decide in advance what students should learn. These critiques, and others, present hurdles to embracing CBE as a viable curricular design strategy.

Integration of Competency-Based Education in the Health Professions

As was noted earlier in this chapter, there has been varied adoption of CBE within the health professions, with medicine, nursing, and social work adopting this curricular structure at varied points in time (Lewis, Rebeschi, and Hunt 2022). While not all disciplines have fully embraced CBE, many are recognizing its role in preparing the next generation of healthcare practitioners. The following sections will provide a brief overview of the current landscape within some of the health professions disciplines.

Medical Education

The development of six clinical competency domains in 1999 by the Accreditation Council for Graduate Medical Education (ACGME) and the American Board for Medical Specialties were one of the first steps in this change. The six domains identified included medical knowledge, patient care, professionalism, interpersonal and communication skills, practice-based learning and improvement, and systems-based practice and system improvement (Desy, Reed, and Wolanskyj 2017). To effectively evaluate and assess these clinical competencies, the integration of clinical skills assessments and milestone exams is becoming more commonplace as academic programs strive to achieve these expectations.

Within medical education, competency-based education has been an ongoing battle as early discussions in the 1990s were met with skepticism (Desy, Reed, and Wolanskyj 2017). However, this began to change in the late 2000s as the ACGME "began restructuring the accreditation system to ensure that assessment and resident promotion depended on these explicit, observable behavioral milestones" (Desy, Reed, and Wolanskyj 2017, 244). This revitalization of the previously developed domains allowed for the implementation of milestones that assessed for explicit behaviors that could be observed.

These milestone markers establish the framework for the competencies and show one's development from novice to expert. Assessed using a descriptive rubric, these milestones are specialty-specific and assess the knowledge, skills, and behaviors needed (Desy, Reed, and Wolanskyj 2017). The integration of the rubric ensures that learner expectations are clearly articulated in a consistent manner. The flexibility of milestones also allows learners to progress at their own pace, providing the freedom Millennial and Gen Z learners desire to drive how they approach learning. "This allows advanced learners to move quickly through requirements leading to early completion and/or other learning opportunities" (Desy, Reed, and Wolanskyj 2017, 246). Furthermore, this ensures that learners requiring more practice or remediation have the time needed to be successful. Benefits associated with milestones-based assessments are that they allow opportunities to provide real-time remediation related to professionalism, emotional intelligence, and behaviors (Desy, Reed, and Wolanskyj 2017). How these milestones assessments are conducted will be discussed later in this chapter.

2003 Institute of Medicine Report and Five Core Competencies

In 2001, the IOM released a report *Crossing the Quality Chasm: A New Health System for the 21st Century* that called for an interdisciplinary summit to explore the reform needed within health professions education to ensure quality patient care and safety (Institute of Medicine Committee on Quality of Health Care in America 2001). The report found that health professions education required an overhaul as it had not remained current with the healthcare systems patient demographics and needs. Specifically, areas of concern focused on the lack of attention to "shifting patient demographics and desires, changing health system expectations, evolving practice requirements and staffing arrangements, new information, a focus on improving quality, or new technologies" (IOM 2003, 1). Using the *Quality Chasm* report as a framework, the committee crafted a new guidance doctrine, the 2003 report *Health Professions Education: A Bridge to Quality*, to support health professions education programs to prepare graduates to meet patient needs. Within the document, they proposed a new vision: "All health professionals should be educated to deliver patient-centered care as members of an interdisciplinary team, emphasizing evidence-based practice, quality improvement approaches, and informatics" (IOM 2003, 3). Furthermore, the committee put forward five competencies for all health professionals designed to meet the needs of healthcare systems: (1) provide patient-centered care; (2) work in interdisciplinary teams; (3) use evidence-based practice; (4) apply quality improvements; and (5)_use informatics (IOM, 2003). These core competencies were identified and shared across health professions disciplines to improve overall patient care and safety (Hodges et al. 2019; IOM 2003).

Nursing Education

The roles in the nursing profession are changing as they are tasked with "emphasizing health equity, improving population health, and caring for an increasingly diverse and aging population" (Lewis, Rebeschi, and Hunt 2022, 1). To prepare the next generation of learners, nursing education must create intentional learning experiences that prepare them for the evolving nature of healthcare. Nursing programs at the undergraduate and graduate levels have guidance documents that outline the core outcomes and their associated expected outcomes which includes the core competencies within the IOM report. In response to the IOM report, the AACN updated the *Essentials* in 2019, which established 10 domains and 8 core concepts that serve as a framework for program and curricular development. Within this framework, there are distinct levels, entry level for baccalaureate and advanced for master's and doctoral programs (Lewis, Rebeschi, and Hunt 2022).

Social Work Education

The 2008 CSWE EPAS marked social work education's transition from focusing on content and structure to focusing on student learning outcomes. As this governing doctrine for baccalaureate and master's level social work programs, this new guidance established the transition from 10 general competencies to 41 specific practice behaviors (McGuire and Lay 2020). In 2015, the updated standards emphasized holistic competence and multidimensional assessment. This redirection encouraged programs to evaluate not just knowledge, values, and skills but also cognitive and effective processes from an integrated approach (CSWE 2015). This revision also saw the implementation of nine interrelated competencies and behaviors. This revised guidance sought to ensure that learners were prepared "to demonstrate the integration and application of the competencies in practice" (CSWE 2015, 6). The 2022 revision maintained the previously identified competencies and behaviors.

Navigating CBE within a Multigenerational Learning Environment

As Sistermans notes, "Integrating competency-based elements into an existing time-based curriculum that caters to cohorts is a complicated, costly intervention" (2020, 683). However, CBE is linked to student-centeredness and self-directedness, which are two areas in which Millennial and Gen Z learners thrive. These generations look to learning environments that are adapted to their own individual needs and strive to engage in learning that is designed to allow them to excel at their own pace. In fact, Millennials and Gen Zs want linkages between what they are learning and real-world practice. They want these experiences to be genuine and relatable to allow them to grow into the professions they have selected for themselves. The integration of CBE within health professions education demonstrates this commitment to ensuring that learners are prepared for practice by creating a curriculum that will provide them with the knowledge, skills, and abilities required to be successful.

One area of concern to be mindful of is that the two generations look at their relationships with their faculty differently. Millennials were raised in a time where assessment driven decisions were made and tend to have sustained the drive needed overtime to push themselves to excel without faculty influence. However, this does not mean that Millennials do not want or expect faculty feedback. Instead, they expect faculty to have clearly articulated learning goals and rubrics so that feedback will be given in a consistent manner. CBE lends itself well to these expectations. Whereas the self-proclaimed self-directed learners, Gen Zs will look beyond their faculty to guide their overall educational experience. They expect and at times demand the integration of technology into their learning environments to support the learning process. Having grown up in a world filled with on-demand information, Gen Zs will supplement what they are learning using technology such as YouTube if it equates to a better learning experience. To adequately support Gen Zs, faculty should be prepared to utilize multiple forms of media within their learning environment to support their students' needs for rapid information delivery. This integration of technology was touched upon in Chapter 5 and will be highlighted later in this chapter.

Millennials and Gen Zs want to feel that they are involved in what they are learning. While Millennials tend to embrace that the institution knows best when it comes to what is being taught, Gen Zs are apt to question information that is provided to them. This calls back to being a product of their environment growing up in a technological heavy world where instant access to information allows them to "check" the information being provided to them by their professor. Unlike Millennials, Gen Zs are not afraid to question authority and consider questioning faculty as their right as it allows them to have control over what they are learning.

As institutions and/or programs look to revitalize their curriculum using competency-based education, it will be important to engage learners within the process to ensure that needs are met. These needs align with the integration of CBE as it allows educators to focus directly on preparing students for future practice without the excess time needed to include extraneous content. Furthermore, the experiential elements of CBE directly correlate to these generations' needs for real-world experiences free from fabricated scenarios.

Competency-based education and clinical skills are closely tied due to the real-world nature of both educational approaches. Clinical skills activities provide the foundation learners need to apply the knowledge, skills, and attitudes required prior to entry into practice. As such, the integration of clinical skills as an assessment approach supports the curricular framework that CBE demands. The next section will examine the role of clinical skills development and the implementation of clinical skills assessments within health professions education.

INTEGRATION OF CLINICAL SKILLS DEVELOPMENT WITHIN HEALTH PROFESSIONS EDUCATION

A key aspect of health professions education is the development of clinical reasoning and skill development (Young et al. 2020). As future healthcare providers, these learners must not only have the knowledge necessary to practice but the hands-on experience required to navigate the varying clinical/practice skills needed for direct patient care. However, these skills must be developed and assessed to ensure that learners are prepared for real-world practice. Often these skills are developed through lab-based skills development courses offered as a component of the traditional classroom-based academic program.

The integration of clinical/practice skills development aligns well with the learning expectations of Millennials and, in particular, Generation Z learners. Gen Zs place greater importance on learning experiences that allow for real-world application and practical learning. The active nature of these experiences and the level of engagement required should support the learning needs of this generation.

Yet, including skills-based training on its own is not enough. These skills must be assessed and aligned with the discipline's required competencies. To effectively assess clinical skills and milestone achievements, it has become common place to integrate objective structured clinical examinations (OSCEs) or simulation-based assessments into health professions curricula (Cruess et al. 2014; Miller 1990). OSCEs are an assessment "of clinical competence in which the components of competence are assessed in a planned or structured way with attention being given to the objectivity of the examination" (Harden 1988, 19). Considered a clinical or practical examination, these performance-based assessments task learners with simulating how they would navigate practice experiences in a safe and controlled environment to allow faculty educators to evaluate student readiness for clinical rotations (Ford and Kleppinger 2020; Harden 1988; McDonough et al. 2015; McGaghie et al. 2014). Specifically, these assessments are designed to focus on what a learner can do and not on what they know. Using these assessments, educators can evaluate learners on one or multiple skill sets, depending on the scenario and assess both process and product. However, before delving into the complexities of creating these types of scenarios, this section will first look at when these types of assessments are warranted.

Medical Education

In 1990, George E. Miller posed the need for an alternative strategy for approaching assessment within medical education. His pyramid-shaped framework included four levels (in order of lowest to highest): level 1—knows (knowledge), level 2—knows how (competence), level 3—shows how (performance), and level 4—does (action). Miller's (1990) new model was designed to incorporate the need for student assessment prior to entering clinical practice, with his most notable focus on the integration of OSCEs into the assessment framework. Miller encouraged his fellow medical educators to think beyond the lower levels of knowledge or competence assessment, noting that they should strive to integrate controlled, practice-based assessments that removed the real patient from the situation until the student had been evaluated more comprehensively. Miller made clear distinctions between the *shows how* and *does* levels; he notes that *shows how* is a performance objective that is ability driven whereas *does* is an action objective that is behavioral driven.

To achieve these higher levels of Miller's pyramid, health professions educators should consider the integration of OSCEs or performance-based assessments prior to transitioning learners into clinical situations. The utilization of OSCEs has been well established in the literature, especially following Ronald Harden's (1988) seminal article outlining what an OSCE is and how this assessment approach aligns with student learning outcomes. While OSCEs had originally been proposed within medical education specifically, Harden (1988) noted that the flexibility of this assessment approach was transferable to other disciplines or subspecialities. Therefore, it is not unusual to see OSCEs or OSCE-like assessments appearing in other health professions areas such as pharmacy and nursing.

Pharmacy Education

In pharmacy education, OSCEs or performance-based assessments (PBAs) are becoming more and more common place as pharmacy educators strive to extend their assessment practices beyond multiple choice exams to holistically evaluate students on their clinical knowledge, reasoning, and skill development (Kristina and Wijoyo 2019). Designed to emulate those offered in medical education, OSCE stations are created to evaluate students' performance effectively and accurately in practice settings. While multiple OSCEs and/or PBAs are being used more frequently in pharmacy education, there continues to be concerns regarding their validity and reliability. Newble and Swanson propose that the low reliability of an OSCE may be attributed to the individual student, "the performance of an examinee on one case or clinical situation is not a good predictor of performance on another case or situation" (1998, 332).

Nursing Education

Nursing education has incorporated OSCEs into their assessment framework since the early 1980s, with one of the first reported instances appearing in South Africa (Goh et al. 2019). Since this date, research shows that OSCEs have been conducted across six continents and 33 countries primarily within academic institutions, but also within hospitals and healthcare organizations and in a limited capacity within some regulatory bodies. However, while OSCEs have been integrated into the assessment framework, often educators have made modifications to the proposed structure Harden and Gleeson (1979) outlined. To evaluate how these modifications impacted the validity and reliability of the assessments, additional research was needed. Goh et al. (2019) conducted a scoping review to examine the existing literature to explore how these changes impacted the validity and reliability of these assessment approaches and found that there was evidence to support OSCEs as valid and reliable methods to assess clinical competence. Furthermore, the findings from this scoping review showed that there was rising interest in OSCEs as a competency-based assessment as it supported educators' evaluations of learners to ensure that they were prepared for patient care and patient safety (Goh et al. 2019). Yet, it is important to note that the authors articulated the importance of not solely relying on OSCEs to evaluate clinical competence as they did not feel that OSCEs were designed to assess the affective and cognitive domains.

Potential Concerns with OSCE Utilization

The integration of OSCEs and PBAs is becoming common practice as the complexities of the healthcare system continue to increase. Yet, we still see some health professions programs wavering in their willingness to include these types of assessments. In the past, educators argued about the appropriateness of using non-practitioners or standardized persons (SPs) as evaluators for clinical practice. However, as far back as Harden (1988) and Miller (1990), it has been noted that non-practitioners when trained appropriately were just as skilled as physicians to evaluate learners.

The cost associated with OSCEs, and PBAs is also often an issue as academic programs must be prepared to cover the expenses associated with creating the appropriate learning and assessment environment to include faculty and SP training and development, and technology upgrades when needed for the simulated environment. Health professions programs must have the space and technology needed to put on these multi-station events. As technology improves and the clinical environment changes, programs must also be prepared to upgrade their simulation environments to include these new resources and to ensure that students are prepared to use the latest technology available to them. With the increasing presence of immersive technologies such as virtual reality (VR) in the classroom, educators must also consider how these new learning resources can be integrated into their learning and assessment environments. The use of immersive technologies in clinical skills development is explored later in this chapter.

Navigating Clinical Skills Development within a Multigenerational Learning Environment

The integration of clinical skills development within health professions education programs serving Millennial and Gen Z learners aligns with the learning preferences of both generations. This alignment is fortuitous as with more and more health professions education programs adopting competency-based education it is likely that the use of simulation experiences will increase (Lewis, Rebeschi, and Hunt 2022). These generations of learners look for opportunities to gain hands-on experiences as it allows them to mimic real-world practice prior to real-world application. Yet, while these generations prefer these types of learning experiences, they may not always see their overarching value if the scenarios do not simulate what they are seeing in the real world. It will be crucial for faculty educators to ensure that the clinical skills and corresponding assessments are designed to immerse these learners into the real-world scenarios they are seeing within their clinical rotations.

Peer feedback and reflection are closely tied to CBE assessments such as case-based and problem-based learning, which drive the development of OSCEs. Utilizing student feedback to refine an academic program will support faculty efforts as they strive to identify authentic assessments that will engage learners while demonstrating the institution's investment in meeting learners where they are. This will also allow faculty to gain a better understanding of effective strategies for integrating opportunities for self-reflection and peer feedback into the curriculum to provide students with the means necessary to express their feelings as well as opportunities to engage with their peers within the learning environment.

Though OSCEs and PBAs have been successfully used, as we transition into generations that are technology savvy, other technologies may need to be explored. In the subsequent sections, immersive technologies are examined to assess their alignment with skills-based learning. Additionally, the pros and cons of these new technologies are discussed.

WHAT ARE IMMERSIVE TECHNOLOGIES?

Immersive technologies create a digital experience utilizing sight, sound, and touch to allow a person to "experience" a virtual, simulated environment. One benefit of immersive technologies is that users can experience an event or environment that may be inaccessible, expensive, or risky to experience in real life. With these technologies, every aspect of a virtual world can be controlled through programming, minimizing the likelihood of unexpected events, unlike real-world experiences. Examples of immersive technologies are virtual reality (VR), augmented reality (AR), and haptics.

Although non-immersive versions of VR do exist, many VR experiences completely immerse the user in the virtual world such that no aspect of the actual physical world can be viewed. This is typically accomplished using a head-mounted display (HMD) such as a Meta Quest or VIVE Pro, although other options exist, including cave systems and Google cardboard. VR is widely used for many applications, including gaming, mindfulness, virtual tours, skill development, educational activities, and treatment of certain health conditions.

AR superimposes a virtual environment onto a physical space such that the user can see both the virtual image and the actual environment simultaneously. Popular applications of AR include Pokémon Go and websites that allow a user to view a piece of furniture that they are considering purchasing in their own home. The benefit of these applications is that they can be experienced at low cost using a smartphone or tablet. More sophisticated (and expensive) AR applications can be experienced using products such as Google Glass or Microsoft HoloLens.

Haptic technologies create tactile sensations, such as pressure, vibration, and movement. Paired with VR or AR, haptics can enhance the user experience by adding this additional element of sensory input, creating a greater degree of immersion and a sense of embodiment (a.k.a., body transfer) which is the feeling of actually inhabiting the body of the virtual avatar. Haptics are found in a wide range of devices, from smartphones and video game controllers to devices like the PHANToM, used in industrial and government research. Haptic gloves like the HaptX Glove can be used to simulate joint stiffness and immobility. A haptic suit, such as the TESLASUIT can be used to simulate sensations over most of the body and for physical rehabilitation and gait training.

Incorporating Immersive Technologies into Health Professions Curricula

Imagine a time when university students in college degree programs are required not only to have a laptop or tablet computer but also a VR headset. With price points starting around $300 per unit at the time of this writing, VR is becoming more and more accessible, making this scenario quite possible, even likely in the next five to ten years. VR is already being used in K–12 schools to teach subjects like science and anatomy and to take virtual field trips (Bailey 2022). As more students are exposed to these technologies early in their education, health professions programs will need to be ready to incorporate these into their curricula. Students will be accustomed to it and even come to expect it. VR has applications far beyond gaming, including patient care, and teaching and learning.

Physical Skill Development and Clinical Decision-Making Using Immersive Technologies

As stated earlier, the incorporation of technology into clinical skills development will be critical to fully engage Millennial and Gen Z learners. As the rate of technological innovation becomes ever more rapid, higher education continues to see the emergence of many new technologies that can augment learning. Immersive technologies are one example and are currently used for the development of skills across many industries. Scalability, the capability of standardizing the clinical experience, and the creation of low-stakes learning environments make these technologies very useful in health professions skills training. VR and AR technologies are commonly used for skill development in hands-on technical skills, such as procedural skills (Bric et al. 2016; Schoeb et al. 2020) and clinical examination (Han et al. 2021). VR has also been used in training for clinical decision-making in trauma scenarios (Harrington et al. 2018). Han and colleagues (2021) tested a program called VRNET (Virtual Reality-based Neurological Examination Teaching Tool) in medical students and found that the Neurologic Physical Examination (NPE) scores were significantly higher in the group that paired VRNET with an SP compared to the group that only used an SP, indicating greater accuracy of assessment among students using the VR-based application.

Because VR can simulate environments that may otherwise be inaccessible or dangerous, it is useful for learning skills in low-stakes situations before needing to perform those skills in a real-world environment where the negative consequences of poor execution are far greater. As mentioned earlier, it is important that these experiences accurately reflect the real-world environments that Gen Z learners are exposed to in experiential settings. Another benefit of incorporating applications that use immersive technologies into the curriculum is that these experiences are easily repeatable, allowing learners to make mistakes, learn from those mistakes, and refine their skills through deliberate practice (Pottle 2019). Drawbacks of the use of immersive technologies include cost of equipment and training, faculty and staff time to implement the activities, and adverse effects of use, such as simulator sickness and eye strain with VR. However, in a VR application used in one college of pharmacy to promote empathy for patients, reports of simulator sickness were very few (8% of participants) and eye strain was reported in only half of users, with half of those reporting experiencing only slight eye strain (Garza et al. 2023).

Communication and Interpersonal Skill Development Using Immersive Technologies

Immersive technologies have been used to train students in best practices for communicating with patients, caregivers, and other healthcare providers. Examples include training on how to respond appropriately to angry patients and caregivers (Fedele 2020; Pan et al. 2016) and how to avoid bias in communication (Banakou, Hanumanthu, and Slater 2016). Reflective listening and non-verbal communication have also been incorporated into VR platforms for communication skills training (Kron et al. 2017). Kron and colleagues (2017) used a VR application to train learners to communicate in intercultural and interprofessional interactions. A subsequent OSCE in advanced communication was used to assess the effectiveness of the training. OCSE communication scores were significantly higher in students randomized to VR compared to those randomized to a computer-based learning module. Students who used VR also reported more positive attitudes and experiences with the application.

Fertleman and colleagues (2018) describe the use of avatars that represent the patients, with health professional trainees playing the part of the provider in interactions that involve dialogue and decision making between provider and patient. Participants reported that they were reminded of their own past experiences in similar situations and felt empathy toward both the provider and the avatar. However, some participants reported uncertainty and overall discomfort during the interaction.

Empathy Development Using Immersive Technologies

Curricula in health professions education often incorporate either case-based activities or experiential opportunities to interact with real patients to promote empathy for patients among learners. The downsides of these approaches are the lack of salience of case-based scenarios and the expense and risk involved with having students interact with real patients. One mechanism to overcome both challenges is to use immersive technologies, like VR, AR, and haptics. These technologies can be used to create experiences designed to promote empathy for patients suffering from chronic health conditions with negative impacts on quality of life. The salience of the patient experience may be greatly enhanced using an immersive technology such as VR, paired with haptic devices to simulate physical impairments associated with chronic disease.

VR has been called the "ultimate empathy machine" (Milk 2015, 03:04) and creates a sense of presence (the feeling of actually being there), plausibility (the feeling that events in VR are actually happening), and embodiment (the feeling that you are actually inhabiting the virtual body). Having students experience firsthand the challenges of participating in activities of daily living due to physical impairments has the potential to impart empathy for these patients. Louie and colleagues (2018) propose that VR can be an effective means to promote empathy among learners due to its ability to allow the user to experience the world through another person's eyes. Additionally, they state that, if effective, VR can be a cost-effective and widely disseminated means of empathy training.

Gillespie and colleagues (2021) found that virtual interactions where the learner played the patient led to an experience of empathy and recognition of areas for improvement in their own communication with patients. They concluded that VR was especially useful to learn more about the patient's lived experiences in the context of social determinants of health. Likewise, Herrera and colleagues (2018) compared a traditional perspective-taking task to VR to promote empathy for unhoused individuals. They found that those who experienced VR had more positive and longer-lasting attitudes toward these individuals and took action to support them at a higher rate compared to participants exposed to the traditional perspective-taking task. Dyer and colleagues (2018) used VR in medical, physician assistant, physical therapy, and nursing students to increase students' empathy for older adults by simulating chronic conditions that older adults often experience, including macular degeneration and age-related hearing loss.

There are potential drawbacks to this approach, however. Researchers have studied the emotional effects of disability simulation on those who experience it and found that it can be a source of psychological distress (Ma and Mak 2022). In addition, it may stigmatize those with disabilities (Silverman 2015). It is vital that health professions programs that are using immersive technologies to promote cognitive empathy for others among learners take special precautions to avoid psychological distress and stigma through education and by ensuring experiences are not painful or shocking, like simulating total blindness and asking learners to navigate the virtual environment. In this example, taking a student who has sight and plunging them into complete darkness without any chance to adapt is not advisable and may have counterproductive consequences. Programs should carefully assess the format and nature of the experience and consider providing a list of counseling resources to participants of these simulations and having debriefing sessions after the experience to discuss any effects, positive or negative, of the learning activity. With a keen awareness of mental health challenges and the toll they can take, Millennial and Gen Z learners would especially appreciate this focus on prevention of distress and availability of resources to address the negative consequences of their learning experiences.

Immersive Technologies for Authentic Assessment

Authentic assessment allows a link between learning and work by situating assessment into environments that are relevant to the real-world workplace (Biggs and Tang 2011). These assessments tend to be well aligned with learning experiences and outcomes and are practical and meaningful for the learner. Immersive technologies, such as AR and VR, lend themselves well to delivery of authentic assessments, as they can simulate a realistic working environment (Looker 2020). As Millennials and Gen Zs value practicality and applicability of learning, use of these technologies for authentic assessment may align well with their learning preferences. It is important to remember that these generations desire clearly articulated expectations of their learning; therefore, it is vital that these technologies are not used indiscriminately and that learning objectives are clearly stated. VR and AR allow the learner to be immersed in realistic scenarios that might otherwise be risky, cost-prohibitive, or inaccessible. For the same reasons, immersive technologies can be useful in CBE where assessments present performance-based tasks or situations (Armstrong, McLaughlin, and Gadarowski 2021).

Use of Immersive Technologies in Millennial and Gen Z Learners

Being accustomed to the ubiquitous use of technology throughout most if not all their lives, learners of the Millennial and Gen Z generations tend to be more highly engaged and invested in their learning when new and interesting technologies are integrated into the curriculum. Student engagement through active learning is widely known to improve learning outcomes. VR, AR, and haptics expose learners to the most cutting-edge technologies and provide experiences that more closely simulate the real-world environment in which they will one day practice compared to traditional methods of simulation.

As mentioned earlier, it is important for educators to collaborate with skilled software developers and use quality equipment to ensure that the virtual environment accurately represents the authentic clinical setting as expected by Millennial and Gen Z learners. Incorporating these technologies into the curriculum can have substantial benefits but must be used with care to avoid negative experiences that may hamper students' learning and/or well-being.

CHAPTER SUMMARY AND CONCLUSION

Millennials and Generation Z learners have a deep appreciation for educational experiences that allow for hands-on learning, real-world application, and critical reasoning skills. The role of clinical skills development is key to ensure that our future healthcare practitioners enter the workforce not only with the knowledge needed but the communication and practice skills necessary for quality patient care. To accomplish this goal, health professions educators must be prepared to identify how their discipline's competencies align with clinical reasoning and practice skills development, and to develop and implement assessments that will ensure that students have achieved the level of practice needed to successful transition into the profession. Use of cutting-edge technologies further engage Millennial and Gen Z learners, potentially improving outcomes of skill development.

Chapter 7 examines how co-curricular experiences help students establish connections within the college and university setting. Furthermore, it describes how student affairs have evolved and how institutions have adapted following generational defining events. An examination of how higher education has adapted to meet the needs and expectations of the younger generation while supporting the Millennial community is also explored.

Chapter 7

Establishing Connection within Co-Curricular Experiences and the Role of Student Affairs within Higher Education

Higher education professionals in co-curricular and student affairs settings are tasked with ensuring that students can access the resources needed to successfully navigate the college environment while cultivating a sense of belonging. This duty can be more complex than one would think, as it requires keeping up with the ever-changing needs of today's college students. In the current landscape, higher education is observing incoming students who are more diverse racially and ethnically, more likely to have substantial employment hours, more likely to wish to attend school part-time, more likely to be parents, and more likely to need online learning (National Association of Student Personnel Administrators [NASPA]: Student Affairs Administrators in Higher Education 2022). How will institutions respond to these demographic changes and work to meet the needs of these students, as opposed to the first-time, full-time traditional students of recent years past? Coupled with learning environment-shaping generational differences of Millennial and Generation Z students, these demographic and enrollment changes bring about a great challenge as institutions work to remain timely and relevant.

This chapter provides a brief overview of the history of student affairs practitioners and examines their role within higher education. Moreover, it will examine how student affairs practitioners support students as they navigate the co-curricular elements of their educational experience. Chapter 7 also defines the co-curricular environment, outlining areas of support, and how the co-curriculum aligns with health professions education.

A BRIEF HISTORY OF THE EVOLVING ROLE OF STUDENT AFFAIRS PRACTITIONERS

The passage of time in higher education has revealed that there are other crucial areas of campus that exist strategically alongside, not just in addition to curricular classroom spaces. NASPA outlined the defining qualities of these co-curricular or student affairs spaces: "Student learning doesn't only happen in a classroom. Opportunities for teaching and development exist everywhere on campus, and it is the responsibility of student affairs professionals to seize these moments and promote positive interactions" (NASPA n.d., para 1). In addition to providing programs and outlets for student learning and development, student affairs practitioners also provide a variety of services and resources for students. Professionals in student affairs realms must work to create environments in which students can thrive personally and professionally during the transitions and challenges that come with being enrolled in an academic institution (Killam and Degges-White 2017).

Student affairs work might involve a focus on student needs, family support, wellness, cost and affordability, academic readiness, support for non-traditional college students, and several other areas of services and programming that work to support students intellectually, emotionally, and socially. To do this work well, a practitioner must collaborate across campus to meet student needs and adapt to change (Killam and Degges-White 2017).

As one considers how practitioners and educators alike will continue to provide adequate services for a new generation of students in an increasingly complex world, it may be helpful to recall that student affairs work is about change, about reconsidering. The field was professionalized on the heels of generation defining events (i.e., World War I and World War II); the end of each revealed the great need for professionals dedicated to intentional student services during ongoing shifts in educational trends and demographics (Long 2012; McClellan and Stringer 2016; Schuh, Jones, and Torres 2017). After World War I, some college student services professional meetings began to gather formally (Long 2012; NASPA 2022). Then, in 1937, *The Student Personnel Point of View* became the guiding and inaugural work of the profession (American Council on Education 1937).

The American Council on Education (ACE) (1937, 1949) described a new "point of view" around the charge for student personnel administrators in the 1930s, and then again in the 1940s. These works established how student affairs and student services work contributed to the value of the institution and furthered the academic mission. The council's 1937 document focused on student development for the betterment of society and developing the student as a whole person, considering achievement, emotion, values, vocation, and relationships (ACE 1937; McClellan and Stringer 2016). The council's 1949 redraft encouraged practitioners to also focus on education for realization of democracy, for understanding and cooperation, and for seeking solutions to social problems (ACE 1949; McClellan and Stringer 2016). As enrollment trends grew following World War II, the American Council on Education (ACE 1949), explored the idea of community and the need for services supporting specialization and graduate programs (NASPA 2022).

As the century went on, the field of student affairs grew and evolved, as the demographics, enrollment, traits, and needs of college students ebbed and flowed. In the 1970s and 1980s, professional organizations and literature began to focus on student learning as an outcome of co-curricular work (NASPA 2022). In 2004, a few short years after yet another horrific and generation defining event (the September 11, 2001, attacks on the United States), student affairs educators and student services professionals were called to yet again "reconsider" their contribution to student learning (Keeling 2004). In *Learning Reconsidered*, student affairs educators were once more encouraged to use the institution's resources to educate and develop the student as a whole person (Keeling 2004). Additionally, practitioners were asked to question their current organizational structures and whether they met the needs of their educational environment. Learning was described as a process that should be student-centered and considered inseparable from a student's overall development (Keeling 2004).

STUDENT AFFAIRS WORK IS ABOUT CHANGE

Throughout the history of the student affairs profession, practitioners have shaped the field by responding to changing demographics and political and world events (Dungy 2018; NASPA 2022). The field of student affairs has centered on the idea of changing with the times and challenging or reconsidering the notions of what has always been accepted by practitioners (Keeling 2004). The entrance of Gen Z into health professions and other professional programs as the world entered a global pandemic reinforced this ongoing need to meet students where they are, understand who they are, and ask what they need to learn and thrive.

Institution-wide and interprofessional approaches will be needed to support students in higher education's changing climate. NASPA asked professionals "to what extent they think their institution is responding to student demographic and enrollment changes" (NASPA 2022, 13). Approximately 33% of respondents agreed that their institutions were adequately dealing with demographic changes, and 45% that their institutions were properly addressing changes in enrollment. Considering the current moment in higher education history and the unique needs of Generation Z students comprising campuses, one must remember that current practices were not necessarily created for these diverse students and professionals who may need unique and varied approaches to address their needs and perspectives. (NASPA 2022)

The current generation of college students has a new set of standards and principles and interestingly are very values-driven in their decision making. In conversation with rising high school seniors, they were asked to discuss their top five priorities in choosing an institution. Surprisingly, the institution's reputation and the quality of their major, while still priorities, were lower on this list than what would have been observed a decade ago. Rather students were more impressed with "the things that institutions are doing, outwardly, to align themselves and their values with the values of the population that they're trying to attract" (NASPA 2022, 13).

Changes Occurring in Real Time

Chapter 3 of this book discussed the anticipation of a "demographic cliff" that will occur in the late 2020s, in which an anticipated decline in the number of high school graduates will also lead to decreases in college applications and enrollment (Grawe 2018, 45). During a webinar presented by the Chronicle of Higher Education in early 2022 titled, *The Demographic Cliff*, a panel of speakers discussed current changes in the higher education market, related to this predicted phenomenon. The panelists acknowledged that without funding, institutions have no mission. As most funding comes from institutional consumers (students), it is imperative to discuss how colleges and universities can continue to create access points for student populations. The speakers noted that practitioners cannot fully rely on pre-pandemic data to predict student trends. However, it can still be insightful to consider the lower birthrates of the Great Recession years and consider the future impacts (Percheski and Kimbro, 2014; Livingston and Cohn 2010). The Pew Research Center's study found that the nation's birth rate grew from 2003 to 2007, and then declined in 2008 and 2009 (Livingston and Cohn 2010). The link to the recession was derived from correlations of state-level birth rate declines to declines in gross domestic product by state and increase in first-time unemployment claims by state. Based on these findings, one can surmise that at times of economic decline, the birthrate will also decline, which will impact institutions of higher education later.

The panelists of the Chronicle's webinar noted observations that lower numbers of undergraduate students are submitting test scores to seek college entry each year. Strategies for recruiting, enrolling, and retaining students may need to shift accordingly. Institutions should look at the demographics of students they are currently enrolling, as well as consider and observe new markets for upcoming academic years. As enrollment demographics continue to shift, it may be necessary to observe, adjust, and observe again. Educators and practitioners must focus not only on new enrollment, but also on retention and persistence. It is not sufficient to focus only on who is being brought into an institution. The speakers noted that the cost of recruiting a new student is greater than the cost of keeping a student who is already enrolled. The speakers also mentioned the importance of getting students engaged on campus, as this is an indicator of persistence (The Chronicle of Higher Education 2022).

As panelists noted, the traditional enrollment funnel has been compromised (Povejsil 2021). Certain demographics of students are not enrolling anymore, at least not at previous rates; if higher education institutions do not find others to enroll, some institutions will not survive. For example, institutions should consider adult learners. If facilities are not open at night, if the registrar and dining options are not open late, it will be difficult to retain these students, even if the courses they need are offered. As practitioners work collaboratively across their institution, they should remember that it requires "a village" to recruit, register, and enroll a class (The Chronicle of Higher Education 2022). Furthermore, administrators should consider who is going to be seeking higher education in the future. Are institutions looking for quick enrollment wins, or are they in the business of supporting students for the long-term (The Chronicle of Higher Education 2022)?

DEFINING CO-CURRICULAR ENVIRONMENTS

Reflecting on the notion that student affairs culture is characterized by responding to change, practitioners must remember that this includes language and the way one communicates concepts regarding the present realities of co-curricular work and priorities. From the origins of student services to dedicated student affairs divisions to the push to emphasize how student affairs work is connected to the curricular experience, it is important to continue to evolve conceptually in how one defines the charge to support students' learning, growth, and development. Roberts (2019) addressed this shift in language in a blogpost titled *Extracurricular vs. Co-curricular*. Roberts (2019) emphasized the differentiation between co-curricular and extracurricular. While "extra" would imply that something is outside or in addition to, student affairs work (particularly the learning and development aspects of this work) is intentionally referred to as "co-curricular," emphasizing partnerships and complementary experiences that allow students to develop holistically, inside, and outside of the classroom. In this sense, co-curricular settings are yet another classroom, filled with practitioners who can guide student learning in their own spaces (Roberts 2019).

Mintz and Rutter defined co-curricular activities as "structured learning activities that complement the formal curriculum" (2016, para 2). The authors continued to state that co-curricular opportunities might include experiential learning, internships/externships, global opportunities, research experiences, and community involvement. The authors continued to emphasize that allowing a focus on the co-curricular ensures that institutions and programs are meeting students where they are. Further, co-curricular practices can be seen as part of the curriculum, when approaches such as flipped classrooms and experiential learning are integrated into the academic experience. Whether outside of or as a component of classroom learning, co-curricular experiences provide alignment across the many ways that students engage and learn (Mintz and Rutter, 2016).

The "Helping Professions"

Perez (2016) explored similarities in what the author referred to as the "helping professions"; examples included student affairs and nursing. In both cases, it is important to help new employees make meaning of their socialization, both professionally and related to self-authorship. Perez presented a new model to help explain how "individuals attempt to make sense of discrepancies or surprises they may encounter during their graduate training" (2016, 36). This type of sense-making is particularly important in helping professions. In education and healthcare fields alike, students are often drawn to the altruism of their future profession, and they go on to study through a combination of theoretical learning and field experience. While in many ways graduates of helping professions will be better prepared through practical application, they may also experience confusion when there is a discrepancy from the classroom to the field (Perez 2016). It is important to provide services to address the need for students to connect theory and practice.

"Do No Harm"—A Concept for Student Affairs and Health Professions Education

Mundell (2022) discussed his evolution as a student affairs practitioner, specifically his interpretation of the concept of nonmaleficence, or *first do no harm*, a concept taught to students of student affairs/higher education and healthcare education alike (ACPA 2020; Council for the Advancement of Standards 2006; Mistry and Rooprai 2020; World Health Organization 2021). Mundell (2022) described that in order to experience growth and development, students must feel safe and must exist in an environment where their well-being is a priority. Practitioners engaged in student affairs work are unable to prevent harm entirely. However, it is crucial that they mitigate harm by prioritizing prevention and appropriate response within a setting that enables students to feel safe and supported. "Working to establish an inherent sense of psychological and physical safety for students is fundamental to our work as student affairs professionals" (Mundell 2022, 19).

Co-curriculum in Health Professions Education

While student affairs or co-curricular offices in health professions schools and programs specifically may not be as clearly defined as those in the broader university, the precedent for supporting student needs, learning, and development in ways that extend past the classroom does exist. The Association of American Medical Colleges (AAMC) maintains an affinity group on student affairs that is concerned with supporting students in areas of admissions, general student affairs, diversity, financial assistance, and student records (AAMC 2023). Similar missions exist in other professions as well. The Office of Student Affairs and Success at a top US nursing school defines its mission as pertaining to support, connections to resources, academic advising, academic program support, recruitment, student records, program compliance, and collaboration with offices coordinating diversity, equity, and inclusion efforts (The Ohio State University College of Nursing, 2023).

In order to see that students within healthcare education environments can function and grow in an environment that promotes their safety and well-being, practitioners and educators have established a variety of services and models to prioritize student support; pharmacy education programs are also an example of how such support has been implemented. Maerten-Rivera et al. (2020) explored how pharmacy programs accredited by the ACPE have implemented co-curriculum models. In 2016, ACPE added a requirement that PharmD programs implement co-curricular activities or "experiences that complement and advance what is taught in the formal didactic and experiential curricula" (Maerten-Rivera et al. 2020, 371). While there is not great consensus on how to define co-curriculum or co-curricular in pharmacy, the requirement suggests that programs should make sure that all students engage in co-curriculum components, and that these opportunities advance learning.

A survey administered by the AACP asked these pharmacy programs what office was responsible for administering the activities of the co-curriculum; the most common response was student affairs or student services departments within the schools. Some schools may have appointed directors for the co-curriculum, a position that could have evolved from previous student affairs or assessment roles within pharmacy schools (Maerten-Rivera et al. 2020). Within the requirement to tie co-curricular activities to learning, several appropriate models were identified. Most of the schools in the study reported that students experienced some level of choice in how they wanted to fulfill their co-curricular requirement, with several schools reporting that this was tied to individual student learning outcomes (Maerten-Rivera et al. 2020).

GENERATIONAL TRAITS AND NEEDS

In order to maintain a focus on student development, it is crucial to understand what drives students; applying a generational lens is one strategy for illuminating students' wants and needs. Even with declining birthrates in the last 15 years (Hamilton, Martin, and Osterman 2021; Kearney and Levine 2021) affecting college enrollment predictions, if a higher percentage of Gen Z students pursue higher education (compared to previous generations), it will be crucial to consider what these students need in and out of a classroom setting. Generational differences already bring about a unique set of needs and preferences; the COVID-19 pandemic brought about an even more nuanced landscape for supporting Gen Z students and rising practitioners.

What Students (and Staff) Need Right Now

Hugus et al. (2021) noted that higher education and student affairs practitioners pivoted to respond to the challenges amid COVID-19 to provide continued support to students and staff, both in-person and virtually. Institutions recognized the need for collaboration and a caring community, but conversely practitioners and students alike found themselves struggling to build relationships in a newly virtual world. Campus members had to be much more intentional about keeping their interactions genuine. The challenges faced during the pandemic caused institutions and practitioners to examine how they should continue to approach student care (Hugus et al. 2021). Institutions have learned to prioritize supporting student mental health, keeping students moving forward, collaboration across varying student support units and among other campus partners, and infusing the unique need to support students into the hiring process. Perhaps above all, the pandemic has taught us the need to prepare for the unplanned (Hugus et al. 2021).

For example, prior to 2020, practitioners felt confident that Generation Z and Millennial students were comfortable with technology, but as the pandemic sent many students, faculty, and staff completely online, institutions learned that the ability to learn and communicate efficiently on these platforms was a new experience. While many campus members, including Millennials and Generation Z individuals, may have possessed digital literacy prior to COVID, there was still a learning curve when it came to proficiency in educational technology (Bergson-Shilcock 2020; Hugus et al. 2021; Wang and Murphy 2020).

What have institutions learned from this digital experience? For one, it is crucial to continually assess digital literacy needs and proficiencies in case there is a need to pivot to a more virtual environment at some point in the future. Also, experiences during and because of the pandemic bring about consideration of issues of flexibility and access; the ability to meet student needs creatively should not be a temporary innovation. Additionally, discussions should continue around how to prioritize engagement versus risk and how to share information in ways that are most impactful for all campus members. Certainly, practitioners and institutions have learned lessons and acquired new perspectives around communication, flexible and efficient policy, and technological tools and uses. Those working with students in curricular and co-curricular settings need to be prepared to take these lessons into the future, for times when students cannot be in-person, of course, but also, in general, to accommodate those learning preferences that have changed (Hugus et al. 2021).

Other Gen Z and Millennial Student Needs in Health Professions Education

Throughout a health professions student's journey, there are many cases in which the need for support and guidance goes beyond academic, extending to a range of personalized needs. As discussed in more depth in Chapter 9, faculty to student mentoring is a crucial relationship within higher education as it supports both the student's educational pursuits and personal growth. Hirsch et al. (2014) studied mentorship among medical students who were intentionally paired with a faculty mentor for research, clinical pursuits, or both. The authors stated that early mentorship activity had a positive impact on choosing a specialty and on ongoing productivity in research activity, as well as on general well-being and future career success.

While mentoring is one piece of the puzzle, the availability of counseling services is vital for Millennial and Gen Z students to support their mental health. Yokotan (2011) discovered that students experiencing grief while under existing academic stress, such as that of being enrolled in a medical school, could endure added emotional consequences. How well medical students coped through their grief process correlated with the type of support they received from their program and specifically its student affairs office.

Chidiac et al. (2018) found that few medical schools in the United States have tobacco cessation programs for students. The authors expressed that this finding was alarming, as many campuses are tobacco free, and many residency programs are implementing new policies prohibiting smokers or tobacco users from entering their programs. Coupled with the lack of cessation programs, few medical programs are making students aware of the career barrier that tobacco usage may present.

Mellman and Paquette (2012) discussed the role of the student affairs dean in medical education stating that this dean should be concerned that their students are both happy and able to perform well academically. Furthermore, the authors felt that student affairs deans should strive to understand the unique traits of medical students enrolled at their institution. To understand these needs, one must consider the cultural and generational implications. Mellman and Paquette (2012) noted that, at that time, Baby Boomer faculty members may have struggled to understand Generation X and Millennial students' priorities, which demonstrates greater loyalty to friends, increased need for balance, and a greater desire for autonomy than faculty may have experienced as students.

Generations have shifted, and the demographics of healthcare education students are now comprised of Millennials and Gen Z. However, Mellman and Paquette's (2012) description of bridging gaps among multigenerational student groups and faculty who are potentially members of additional generational groups still stands today. Growing up, Millennials experienced the rise of the internet; constant access to communication; overly busy schedules, with an emphasis on involvement and participation; protective and involved parenting; and as a result of busy schedules, were catered to when scheduling conflicts arose at school or in activities. Due to this upbringing, Millennials in medical school or other healthcare education environments may demand quick communication when issues arise, ease of access to professors and resources, and a personal approach to guidance from their mentors (Mellman and Paquette 2012).

An important part of fostering more diverse environments and cohorts within health professions education involves educating students and other campus members about threats to diverse and equitable climate. Sukhera and Walting (2018) presented a six-point framework designed to help faculty and staff as they integrate the recognition of and efforts to overcome implicit bias in health professions education. The framework involves education that encourages perspective-taking, empathy, and a social approach to meaningful dialogue. The authors suggest discussing topics such as what is implicit bias; how can implicit bias impact clinical and patient outcomes; and how to become more aware of where it exists and ways to mitigate its effects (Sukhera and Walting 2018).

GEN Z AND MILLENNIAL EMPLOYEES IN THE HIGHER EDUCATION/ STUDENT AFFAIRS WORKPLACE

As the prominent generation of current student affairs professionals continues to shift, viewpoints in workplaces and in the field in general have shifted as well (Perkins and Herring 2021). This is evident in supervisor/employee interactions, as well as in professionals' trajectories. New professionals in student affairs and co-curricular work are mostly Zillennials, (roughly born between 1992 and 1998) (Perkins and Herring 2021). Supervising these new professionals may be similar to supervising or mentoring undergraduate and professional students, as certain common Gen Z traits are evident in both. For example, there is a need for external feedback exhibited by both students and Zillennial employees in order to develop.

It is also important for professionals in co-curricular settings to remember that their staffs are bridging generations. An effective professional setting will require supervisors to lead across generations, from the staff members they motivate to the students they support. Perkins and Herring ask, "What does it mean to approach supervision when professionals run the gambit of generations and are increasingly diverse in other ways, yet our departmental and institutional leaders are largely still Baby Boomers and the oldest members of Generation X?" (2021, 74). This cross generational leadership may require supervisors to challenge their ideas around professional development and leadership so that they can meet employees' unique generational needs (Brown 2022; Giancola 2006; Perkins and Herring 2021). While Perkins and Herring's (2021) article is more about supporting staff members, their sentiment could be a good commentary on the range of generational influences that impact the landscape of higher education institutions at the current moment.

While it is easy to focus efforts at leading across generations on the need to understand Generation Z, it would be remiss to exclude consideration of the fact that Millennials are still the largest part of the US workforce (Brown 2022; Perkins and Herring 2021), including most higher education professions. Older Millennials are still actively entering middle and senior management roles. If higher education and student affairs practitioners are to support traditionally aged Generation Z students as well as non-traditional aged students from several generational cohorts, educators must consider the traits of Millennials that still comprise many roles across campuses.

HEALTH PROFESSIONS AND STUDENT AFFAIRS: A PRACTITIONER IS ALSO A STUDENT

Student affairs environments and health professions education settings are similar in that the line between student and professional is somewhat blurred. Traditional student affairs divisions and offices employ many entry-level full-time professionals who may be relatively close in age to the graduate and undergraduate students they supervise and support. Similarly, within student affairs settings, graduate students grow professionally, as future full-time practitioners in their field, often in internships and assistantships allowing them to hold a supervisory role with undergraduate students. Additionally, some undergraduate students in these spaces serve in student leadership roles designed to help them develop many of the same capacities.

Health professions education follows a similar pattern, in that the student does not become a professional and a leader overnight. Students follow a path of experiential learning, in which they work alongside mentors, gradually taking on additional responsibility and leadership tasks. Even when one has achieved degree completion within health professions education, their journey as a learner is often far from over. These new professionals may embark on residencies and fellowships to continue refining their work in their field, as both a student and a practitioner. Ultimately, the goal is to become one who fully identifies with and has taken on the role of a member of their profession. However, the cycle of teaching and learning is embedded throughout one's career.

CHAPTER SUMMARY AND CONCLUSION

Since student affairs work and health professions education are both about growth and development, it is a natural assumption that the co-curricular elements of a healthcare education setting are especially vital to meeting the needs of the whole student. As noted in *The Compass Report*, "the shifting demographics and expectations of today's students highlight the need to focus on their mental health and basic needs, technology and online engagement, learning inside and outside the classroom, and cross-institutional collaboration" (NASPA 2022, 13). Student affairs work was created for change, and the present climate is one in which much change is on the horizon.

On the heels of the COVID-19 pandemic and in anticipation of the demographic cliff, it is reasonable to predict that students will need increased and enhanced support. With heavy workloads and unique burdens, health professions students are no exception. Offices that coordinate student affairs and student services, within the greater campus and within health professions schools specifically, must continue to increase offerings in line with current needs and generational trends. In order to navigate the changing climate, students and young professionals from the Millennial and Generation Z cohorts will need provisions focused on mental health, accommodations, diversity, flexibility, balance, and holistic well-being.

Higher education, experiential learning, and workplace environments must adapt so that younger generations feel that their needs are met, while also providing encouragement to Millennial and Gen Z community members to work with members of other generations to capitalize on shared values and complementary strengths. It will be the work of the co-curricular to see that students (and future professionals/practitioners) develop and grow both in and out of the classroom, within these ever-changing contexts.

Chapter 8 examines the role of interprofessional education (IPE) and interprofessional teams within multigenerational populations. The integration of IPE into health professions education aligns with the diverse nature of healthcare and prepares students to learn about and with others who will be working alongside them upon entry into practice. This chapter examines the role of IPE in a variety of educational settings and will provide guidance regarding the development and implementation of these programs.

Chapter 8

Creating a Team within Interprofessional Education with Multigenerational Student Populations

The World Health Organization (WHO) defines interprofessional education (IPE) as occurring "when students from two or more professions learn about, from, and with each other to enable effective collaboration and improve health outcomes" (2010, 10). In their report, *Framework for Action on Interprofessional Education and Collaborative Practice* (hereafter referred to as the WHO *Framework*), the WHO recognized IPE as a critical component of education for all health professions (World Health Organization [WHO] 2010). Four competencies have been identified by the Interprofessional Education Collaborative (IPEC) to guide teaching of interprofessional collaboration: values and ethics, roles and responsibilities, communication, and teamwork (Interprofessional Education Collaborative [IPEC] 2016). These are depicted in Figure 8.1 and described in detail later in the chapter.

At the core of IPE is collaboration between members of the healthcare team, leading to improved patient outcomes. Fragmentation of health systems globally results in unmet patient care needs, necessitating a team-based approach to patient care to address those needs. Such an approach utilizes a team of professionals who know how to optimize the differing skills of team members to provide quality care to address a wide range of health conditions, coordinating their efforts to work collaboratively with patients and caregivers to achieve their desired healthcare goals (WHO 2010). A team-based approach to care has been shown to improve health outcomes and reduce healthcare costs through increased access to care; decreased patient complications, hospital length of stay, and readmission rates; reduced incidence of medical errors; and improved patient satisfaction (WHO 2010; Will, Johnson, and Lamb 2019). In the WHO *Framework*, the authors make

Competency 1: Values and Ethics	• Work with individuals of other professions to maintain a climate of mutual respect and understanding
Competency 2: Roles/Responsibilities	• Use the knowledge of one's own role and those of other professions to appropriately assess and address the healthcare needs of patients and to promote and advance the health of populations
Competency 3: Interprofessional Communication	• Communicate with patients, families, communities, and professionals in health and other fields in a responsive and responsible manner that supports a team approach to the promotion and maintenance and the prevention and treatment of disease
Competency 4: Teams and Teamwork	• Apply relationship-building values and the principles of team dynamics to perform effectively in different team roles to plan, deliver, and evaluate patient/population-centered care and population health programs and policies that are safe, timely, efficient, effective, and equitable

Figure 8.1 Interprofessional Education Collaborative Competencies for IPE.
Source: Adapted from Interprofessional Education Collaborative, 2016.

the distinction between teams that simply work together and agree to utilize their skills toward a common goal, compared to teams consisting of members with complimentary skills who collaborate to develop a shared understanding where no such understanding previously existed, creating synergy in the delivery of patient care (WHO 2010). It is the latter that is critical to addressing the patient care challenges of a fragmented healthcare system. This shared understanding should include not only recognition of the diverse skills and expertise contributed by individual group members but should also honor generational differences that are likely to exist.

IPE is an important mechanism for preparing health professionals to practice in these collaborative teams. IPE bridges local health needs and collaborative practice to optimize health services and improve overall health outcomes within the context of health and education systems. Documented benefits of IPE to learners include improvements in knowledge, skills, attitudes, and competency in collaboration (Abu-Rish et al. 2012; Reeves et al. 2016). If conducted effectively, IPE results in respect for other members of the healthcare team, reduces negative stereotypes, and supports patient-centered care (WHO 2010). IPE creates a "collaborative practice-ready" workforce by training learners to work together in collaborative teams, with the ultimate goal of improving healthcare outcomes through system efficiencies and cost-effectiveness (WHO 2010, 7). As stated in the WHO *Framework*,

> Interprofessional education and collaborative practice can play a significant role in mitigating many of the challenges faced by health systems around the world.

> Now is the time to act, to implement these strategies which have the potential to transform health-care delivery, strengthen health systems, and ultimately improve health outcomes. (2010, 41)

An environmental scan by Rodger et al. on behalf of the WHO, examining geographic areas where IPE is utilized and how it is conducted, found that students of the following health professions participate in IPE around the globe: audiologists, community health workers, dentists/oral hygienists, nurses/midwives, nutritionists, occupational therapists, pharmacists, physicians, physician assistants, physiotherapists, podiatrists, psychologists, social workers, speech pathologists, and others (Rodger et al. 2010). Survey respondents, individuals who work with health professions students in any of the 193 WHO member states, indicated that IPE was delivered in various formats and settings in their learning programs, including lectures/presentations by teaching faculty, written cases, small group discussion, interactions with simulated patients, and practice-based patient care as part of a healthcare team. However, three-quarters of survey respondents indicated that their students received less than six months of IPE across their learning program, and more than two-thirds reported that their programs did not provide staff training for development and delivery of IPE.

IPE may be a student's first experience with collaborating with team members of other generations (North Arizona University Teaching Academy 2016). As has been discussed in previous chapters, teaching and learning across generations can present challenges, given the varied learning preferences and values held by members of different generations. Unfortunately, educators often assume that students know how to navigate differing generational viewpoints and approaches to teamwork. A need exists to advance IPE in programs that currently lack a substantial IPE component, and resources for faculty development in this area are needed. This chapter will provide a brief history of IPE, and then focus on guidance for educators to effectively develop and implement IPE in groups of learners that span different generations.

EVOLUTION OF IPE IN HEALTH PROFESSIONS

Driven by the rising prevalence of co-morbidities and greater complexity of specialty care, healthcare is increasingly delivered by a team of professionals covering a wide range of disciplines whereby all members of healthcare teams serve a role in positively impacting patient care (Babiker et al. 2014). With increasing global demand for improvements in quality of care, and as clinical teams become a more critical factor influencing health outcomes, greater emphasis has been placed on a patient-centered teamwork approach. Accordingly, health professions education began to recognize the importance of building skills in teamwork and communication among members of healthcare teams. The National Academy of Medicine identified five core principles of team-based patient care that support effective healthcare teams: (1) shared goals, (2) clear roles, (3) mutual trust, (4) effective communication, and (5) mutual processes and outcomes (Smith et al. 2018).

In 1987, the Centre for the Advancement of Interprofessional Education (CAIPE), based in the United Kingdom, was established to "support and promote interprofessional education and practice" (Dickie 2016, 1). Establishment of the CAIPE coincided with publication of a report by the WHO, *Learning Together to Work Together for Health* (WHO 1988). Additionally, an increasing focus on medical errors and deficiencies in the healthcare system regarding teamwork and communication arose with the publication of *To Err Is Human: Building a Safer Healthcare System*, a report by the IOM, a component of the National Academy of Sciences in the United States (Kohn, Corrigan, and Donaldson 2000). This seminal report focused on patient safety and ways to reduce the high incidence of medical errors and subsequent patient deaths. It was a striking call to action for healthcare systems and led to a wide range of initiatives to improve healthcare quality in the United States. These events sparked increased interest among health education programs, and the IPE movement began to pick up momentum.

Team Science

Likewise, team science, where a team of researchers from various disciplines collaborates on a single research project to address problems in healthcare, has grown in importance. Accordingly, a team science approach has become a focus of agencies that fund healthcare research, creating an even greater emphasis on building interdisciplinary teams in the academic setting (Little et al. 2017). To date, team science has developed momentum along a separate path from IPE. However, a systematic review of the literature established that team science is a component of the larger domain of interprofessional collaborative practice, and the authors recommend that team science be incorporated into IPE initiatives "in order to bring together health professions education, clinical practice, and health sciences research training and practice" (Little et al. 2017, 21).

The work of collaborative research teams also provides challenges when membership crosses generations. In an article published in *Science* magazine titled "From Selfies to Selfless: Managing Multigenerational Teams," Levine describes the keys to leading such teams as consisting of (1) flexible, open lines of communication; (2) understanding and aligning various generational cultures; and (3) individualizing solutions for managing team members (2017). The author also warns against stereotyping team members based on generational membership, as discussed in Chapter 1 of this book (Levine 2017).

One Health

Yet another movement that has further contributed to the formation of IPE programs is the One Health movement that emerged in 2004, described as a global strategy incorporating a holistic, transdisciplinary, and multisectoral approach to health (Courtenay et al. 2015; Destoumieux-Garzon et al. 2018). The American Veterinary Medical Association defines One Health as "the integrative effort of multiple disciplines working locally, nationally, and globally to attain optimal health for people, animals, and the environment" (American Veterinary Medical Association 2022). Increased globalization, influenced by population growth, industrialization, and geopolitical problems have contributed to increasing threats resulting from environmental or zoonotic sources (Destoumieux-Garzon et al. 2018). The One Health movement proposes to address these threats through a collaborative interdisciplinary approach, encompassing human health, animal health, and environmental health.

IPE PREPARES HEALTH PROFESSIONS STUDENTS FOR PRACTICE

IPE has been around for many years, with some sources citing IPE programs as far back as the 1960s. Given the trends described above, IPE began to really take off in the early to mid-2000s and has grown in influence and impact over the subsequent two decades. A 2007 review of 21 studies evaluating the effectiveness of IPE demonstrated that IPE increased knowledge and skills necessary for collaboration and was generally well-received by participants (Hammick et al. 2007). A 2008 Cochrane review evaluating effectiveness of IPE was also conducted, with four of six studies showing positive impacts on delivery of care, patient satisfaction, collaborative team behavior, and reduced error rates, with two studies showing no impact (Reeves et al. 2008). A more recently conducted systematic review included 25 new studies to add to the 21 found in Hammick and colleagues' 2007 review, for a total of 46 studies (Reeves et al. 2016). Results of this review demonstrated increasingly positive outcomes of IPE, further supporting its effectiveness as an educational approach, in particular, improvements in attitudes, knowledge, and skills of student learners.

Classroom-based IPE

IPE has been delivered in many different modalities and in different settings. Early IPE experiences were often didactic in nature. For example, students from multiple health professions programs might take an ethics course together. Students in such a course would benefit from the sharing of differing perspectives during large group discussions around case studies. Classroom-based IPE is still widely used and can be an effective modality. A systematic review examining effectiveness of classroom-based IPE programs demonstrated improvements in collaboration and students' attitudes toward learning, and qualitative data suggested both educational and social gains with classroom-based IPE (Vuurberg et al. 2019). The most frequently used training formats for classroom-based IPE were lectures, small group activities, including simulation settings, and e-learning materials. As discussed in Chapter 5, both Millennials and Gen Zs prefer stimulation in the classroom and value hands-on experiences, necessitating the incorporation of active learning strategies and approaches that allow the use of technology to maintain student engagement.

Experiential IPE

Clinical settings for IPE are also common. For example, 55% of US pharmacy schools surveyed reported that IPE was occurring in introductory clinical rotations, termed Introductory Pharmacy Practice Experiences (IPPE) (Grice et al. 2018). IPE has been delivered as service-learning experiences, as described by Bridges and colleagues (2011). They demonstrate how one school of medicine and science tasked first-year students from seven different health professions with working with community partners to carry out a community-service project. Another setting in which IPE is frequently conducted is in experiential learning sites in patient care settings. Among medical education programs, experiential IPE has been shown to result in positive student attitudes toward learning, enjoyment of learning, and a better understanding of the nurse's role in patient care (Walmsley, Fortune, and Brown 2018). A subset of these experiences occurs in the context of home visits for volunteer patients and caregivers. Students are tasked with taking a thorough family history and providing a report on what occurred at each home visit. In lieu of conducting IPE among real patients, some programs utilize simulation, including manikins, standardized persons, or game-based simulations. More information about the use of simulation in health professions education can be found in Chapter 6.

With the evolution of team-based care and the rise of IPE, terminology has also evolved. Though often used interchangeably, the terms "interdisciplinary" and "multidisciplinary" have distinct meanings. Multidisciplinary teams are groups of professionals with varied skill sets and areas of expertise, providing greater breadth of services, but mostly operating independently of and parallel to one another; whereas interdisciplinary teams consist of members with varied skills and expertise who work collaboratively to reach a common goal, integrating each professional's knowledge into the plan of care (American Hospital Association [AHA] 2020). Other terms, such as transdisciplinary, multiprofessional, interprofessional, transprofessional, shared learning, common learning, collaboration, common studies, joint training, joint learning, and joint studies have entered the IPE lexicon (Ford and Gray 2021). CAIPE uses the phrase "interprofessional education" to encompass all of these in both academic (pre-qualification) and work-based (post-qualification) settings (Ford and Gray 2021).

IPE has been endorsed by many accrediting bodies for health professions education, including the Liaison Committee on Medical Education (LCME), Accreditation Council for Pharmacy Education (ACPE), Accreditation Commission for Education in Nursing (ACEN), Commission on Dental Accreditation (CODA), and many others, spanning a broad array of health professions programs (Health Professions Accreditors Collaborative [HPAC] 2019). Six accrediting bodies came together in 2014 to create the Health Professions Accreditors Collaborative (HPAC) to formalize interactions across organizations and serve as a platform for sharing information and problem-solving. In 2019, 24 accrediting organizations endorsed a guidance document on IPE drafted by the HPAC in collaboration with the National Center for Interprofessional Practice and Education (NCIPE) at the University of Minnesota, making IPE well-established and accepted by educational programs for a vast majority of health professions (HPAC 2019).

STRATEGIES AND CHALLENGES FOR IMPLEMENTATION OF IPE IN HEALTH EDUCATION CURRICULA

Mechanisms that shape IPE are outlined in the WHO *Framework* and categorized as "educator mechanisms" and "curricular mechanisms" (WHO 2010, 38). Educator mechanisms include identifying champions, institutional support, managerial commitment, shared objectives, and staff training. Curricular mechanisms include adult learning principles, assessment, compulsory attendance, contextual learning, learning outcomes, logistics and scheduling, and managing program costs. Based on this report, Rodger et al. outlined the following evidence-based practices for IPE (2010, 487):

1. IPE should be a mandatory component of every health professional's education.
2. IPE should be offered based on explicit learning outcomes that are made clear to both staff and students.
3. IPE should be assessed with respect to what students are intended to learn.
4. IPE should be offered by trained facilitators who have received staff development in this area.
5. IPE should be evaluated for both process and outcomes.

Competencies for Interprofessional Education

As mentioned previously, the IPEC revised its list of core competencies for IPE in 2016. The original collaborative came together in 2009 and consisted of six national associations of schools of health professions representing dentistry, nursing, medicine, osteopathic medicine, pharmacy, and public health. As of 2016, IPEC had expanded to include nine new institutional members representing podiatry, physical therapy, occupational therapy, psychology, veterinary medicine, optometry, allied health, social work, and physician assistants. The complete list of IPEC competencies is contained in Figure 8.1.

Other commonly utilized sources for guidance on implementation of IPE in health professions education are the *CAIPE Interprofessional Education Guidelines 2017* (Barr et al. 2017) and the *CAIPE Interprofessional Education Handbook* (Ford and Gray 2021). Creation of competency-based outcomes relevant to the disciplines involved is an important step in the development of effective IPE programs. Ford and Gray (2021) describe three types of competence: common competencies, which are common across all professions; complementary competencies, which are important to one profession but complement the competence of another profession; and collaborative competencies, which allow team members of different professions to work collaboratively and effectively with one another.

Learning Theories and Approaches That Shape Development and Implementation of IPE

Ford and Gray (2021) explain that an underpinning of theoretical frameworks helps to ensure effectiveness of IPE learning opportunities. Theories may include those that explain individual behavior (e.g., theories on emotional intelligence), those that explain group behavior (e.g., theories about group member roles, shared social capital, and belonging), and learning theories (e.g., experiential learning theory). Successful IPE generally follows student-centered learning approaches and utilizes trigger material to establish concrete experience, reflective observation through discussion, and abstract conceptualization, and then utilize active experimentation as a team to determine how learning will impact their future practice. Further discussion of the application of Kolb's Experiential Learning Theory (Kolb, Boyatzis, and Mainemelis 2014), for example, can be found in Chapter 9 in the context of experiential learning. Potential learning approaches are outlined by Barr et al. (2017) and include problem-based learning, case-based learning, collaborative inquiry, appreciative inquiry, observation-based learning, experiential learning, reflective learning, simulated learning, continuous quality improvement, and others. Selection of these approaches should consider the unique needs of Millennial and Gen Z learners described in Chapter 5, such as use of technology in the learning environment, modeling of behavior, and hands-on experiences.

Planning and Delivery of IPE Learning Experiences

In keeping with the spirit of collaborative practice, planning, and delivery of IPE programs should likewise be collaborative, with planning team members having equal status and involvement (Ford and Gray 2021). Development of interprofessional aims should accommodate both "interprofessional" and "uniprofessional" (of a single profession) needs of learners from all professions and across generations. The planning team should engage with differences across disciplines that result from use of varying terminology and underlying philosophies to determine how the three essential components of IPE, learning *with*, *from*, and *about* other professions, will be accomplished. This involves consideration of what uniprofessional skills each group of learners brings to the team, how balanced interaction will allow them to learn from one another, and how to work together and learn about one another to achieve learning outcomes related to changes in attitudes, knowledge, or behavior. Developers of new IPE programs are encouraged to learn from those who have experience in IPE development and to compare and contrast various programs in different contexts and settings to determine the best fit for their own programs (Barr et al., 2017).

It is also of vital importance to foster an environment of inclusivity, avoiding alienation of students from any particular health profession. Ford and Gray (2021) state that materials used to promote IPE in an institution "should avoid, as far as possible, language and assumptions that imply bias toward certain professions, for example, if the publicity is aimed at attendees from social care, then the terms such as 'client' or 'service user' as well as 'patient' should be used" (Ford and Gray 2021, 13). Inclusive teaching is especially important in this context, given differing educational backgrounds, ages (and thus generational membership), and competency levels of learners.

Challenges to IPE program development include differing practice backgrounds, theoretical orientation, and preferred learning styles of educators, as well as differences in course length, timing, and structure when attempting to introduce IPE across two or more courses from differing disciplines. Particularly challenging are varying student schedules, especially in the case of lock-step curricula with little flexibility in the sequence and timing of which required courses are taken. These challenges necessitate agreement among parties at the outset regarding when, where, and how to introduce IPE.

Necessary Components and Qualities of IPE Learning Experiences

Barr et al. (2017) propose that responsibility for learning in an IPE environment rests on the group as much as it does on individual team members, making the team a community of practice. Learning together can prepare participants for collaborative practice by mitigating the promotion of prejudice, stereotypes, and rivalry, and fostering mutual awareness, trust, and respect. The authors also state that members should "explore how each of them can contribute to a process of cooperative, cyclical, iterative, reflective and socially constructed learning, towards the resolution of conflicts, and the development of insight, understanding and skills" (Barr et al. 2017, 4). Structured learning activities that require interaction should be implemented among small interprofessional groups (Ford and Gray 2021). These activities should allow every participant to play an active role and to contribute their unique expertise to the activity.

Group members should establish shared goals and treat one another with mutual respect, acknowledging their differences. IPE prepares learners to go beyond simple cooperation to embrace a "planned, purposeful, concerted, and sustained endeavor within a defined legal and policy context to ensure comprehensive provision of quality care which transcends demarcations between professions, between practice settings, and between organisations [*sic*]" (Barr et al. 2017, 5). IPE facilitators should recognize the importance of interaction and group identity, countering the natural tendency for group members to gravitate toward those from their own disciplines (Ford and Gray 2021). Because of the strong need for development of group identity, members should be organized into small teams with balanced numbers of representatives from each profession who stay together for the duration of the activity, allowing team bonds to form. It is also important to allow sufficient time for introductions and for members to get to know one another before learning activities begin. This is especially true for team members of different generations.

As described previously, IPE can occur in a classroom, community, or clinical setting. In regard to what Ford and Gray refer to as "space and place" (2021, 12), neutral territory is recommended so that all group members feel at home and comfortable in the venue. Classroom IPE settings should be carefully chosen to meet the complex needs of the learners. With 5–8 being the most ideal group size, the facility should have tables to accommodate groups with room for comfortable discussion among team members and space for facilitators to circulate freely. IPE in the community or clinical setting provides opportunities for learners to engage in real-world immersive experiences and anticipate situations they may see in their own future clinical practice (Barr et al. 2017). It requires coordination between educational institutions and community and practice sites to ensure high-quality professional and interprofessional experiences, learner satisfaction, and achievement of learning objectives. For a more detailed discussion, Chapter 9 explores experiential learning and the impact of real-world experiences on student development.

Assessment Practices in IPE

As stated previously, IPE should be assessed with respect to the intended student learning outcomes (Rodger et al. 2010). Student learning in IPE can be assessed in a variety of ways. Assessment of learning may be accomplished through reflections, learning logs, portfolios, or performance-based exams (Barr et al. 2017). Feedback elicitation between activities and at the end of the session is helpful to maintain a learner-centered approach. Evaluation of the learning activity should occur at the conclusion of the event to assess learning outcomes, interprofessional content, engagement, potential to impact learner behaviors and outcomes of care. Findings from the evaluation should then be used to refine the experience, creating a continuous quality improvement feedback loop.

The NCIPE provides tools for assessment of student learning and other outcomes of IPE (National Center for Interprofessional Practice and Education [NCIPE] n.d.). These tools measure a variety of domains, including but not limited to teamwork; attitudes, values, and beliefs; behaviors and skills; patient, provider, and trainee satisfaction; and organizational environment or culture. Multiple methods of measurement are available, including self-report (surveys, questionnaires, self-ratings), observation (rubrics, rating tools, or 360-degree feedback), and use of recording templates, such as a chart audit. Many of these tools are available for free through open access on the NCIPE website (2022).

One widely used tool is the Student Perceptions of Interprofessional Clinical Education Revised (SPICE-R), which is a self-report survey that measures health professions students' perceptions related to IPE and interprofessional collaborative practice (Dominguez et al. 2015). Domains include interprofessional teamwork and team-based practice, roles and responsibilities, and patient outcomes from collaborative practice. Another IPE assessment tool is the Performance Assessment Communication and Teamwork Tools Set (PACT), which includes five instruments: two self-report pre-post assessments and three observational rating tools (Chiu 2014). These instruments measure team structure, leadership, situation monitoring, mutual support, and communication, the five domains of the Team Strategies and Tools to Enhance Performance and Patient Safety (TeamSTEPPS™) model (King et al. 2008).

Effective Facilitation of IPE Learning Activities

IPE facilitators should be present to set the scene, manage logistics, ensure participants understand the task, and facilitate group discussion when needed (Ford and Gray 2021). Their role in IPE is not to deliver information but to support reflective learning. Having skilled facilitators with credibility drawn from expertise, who are sensitive to differences among professions, and who use an inclusive approach is also important. This often requires facilitators to step out of their own professional roles and act as a "generic professional" (Ford and Gray 2021, 15). It also requires that they be alert to any barriers or tensions related to hierarchy, status, and differing philosophies and approaches to care. Facilitators of various professions should model collaboration and effective interprofessional interactions, working as equals, having mutual respect for one another's expertise, and demonstrating how the different professions complement one another. Skills that are important for facilitators to possess are active listening, ability to effectively manage difficult group dynamics, understanding of adult learning theories, and skills to support others to learn. Training and support of institutional resources are vital to faculty development in both facilitation and teaching of IPE. Centers such as the NCIPE provide train-the-trainer programs and other faculty development resources.

Team Dynamics in IPE

Teamwork is approached very differently by Millennials compared to Generation Z. As described in Chapters 1 and 2, Millennials, though sometimes known as the "Me Generation," are generally quite collaborative and value peer interaction, while Gen Zs prefer to work in groups that operate as individual members, dividing the work and coming back together at the end of a project to put it all together (Seemiller and Grace 2016). Likewise,

Millennials tend to be more rule-governed and less likely to question authority, while Gen Zs tend to be more accepting and inclusive of group members compared to older generations (Howe and Strauss 2003; Shatto and Erwin 2016; Wilkins 2021). These varied approaches and affinity for teamwork can lead to challenges when operating as part of an interprofessional team. Cox and Holloway list four activities critical to the successful operation of multigenerational teams: communication, inclusion, trust, and conflict resolution (Cox and Holloway 2011).

Moore, Everly, and Bauer contend that open communication is the cornerstone of effective teamwork when teams are multigenerational (2016). Preferences for mode of communication differ across generations, meaning that skilled group leaders might use multiple methods of communication using different channels to reach members from different generations, demonstrating respect for all members. Refer to Chapters 1 and 2 for a detailed description of differences in communication styles and preferences across Millennials and Gen Z.

Promotion of inclusivity among the team requires efforts to empathize and identify with working styles of fellow team members of other generations and appreciate what each group can contribute to the team. As mentioned in the section above on Effective Facilitation of IPE, it is vital that facilitators ensure that all voices are heard and that team members of all participating health professions feel welcome and included. This requires mutual awareness and understanding of the skills that each profession contributes to the group. Likewise, awareness and appreciation of generational differences can help foster this culture of inclusivity. Given that Millennials and Gen Zs are the most diverse generations, a need also exists to ensure inclusivity among learners from various underrepresented groups (Howe and Strauss 2003; Wilkins 2021).

Also mentioned earlier in the chapter, trust among team members is particularly important on a patient care team where the aim is to provide competent, safe, and compassionate care (Moore, Everly, and Bauer 2016). According to Douglas et al., "When team trust exists, team members are willing to admit mistakes, share their weaknesses, and express their concerns without fear of retaliation" (2015, 11). Trust-building can be supported by asking for and offering help and giving feedback.

An environment of open communication, inclusivity, and trust facilitates effective conflict resolution (Moore, Everly, and Bauer 2016). Effective teams develop approaches that frame conflict as beneficial and appreciate the varied generational approaches to conflict resolution. Inability to effectively resolve conflicts or avoiding them altogether can lead to mistrust and a dysfunctional team dynamic (Douglas et al. 2015). Douglas et al. encourage the adoption of formal signed team agreements or contracts to explicitly lay out expectations to avoid miscommunication and misunderstanding (2015). These formal agreements communicate respect for differing viewpoints across generations, create a sense of unified commitment, and help establish accountability.

Faculty and Preceptor Development for Delivery of IPE

Faculty and preceptor training and development is critical for the effective delivery of IPE in health professions education. As previously mentioned, NCIPE, in collaboration with HPAC, developed a guidance document for development of IPE programs (HPAC 2019). This guidance calls for a systematic approach at the institutional level and possible realignment of resources to support the development of IPE programs. Related to this, faculty must be given protected time for program development and IPE-focused faculty development opportunities. Faculty development programs should include information on the preferences and behaviors of both Millennial and Gen Z learners outlined in this chapter and the subtle nuances that distinguish them and provide practical strategies to maximize their learning in IPE settings.

Silver and Leslie (2017) describe a framework for IPE faculty development based on best practices in faculty development and continuing interprofessional education. The authors posit that consideration must be given to all three levels of an organization: the micro- (learner, educator, and learning context), meso- (leadership and administrative), and macro-level (accreditation and institutional structures) when developing an IPE curriculum. At the micro-level, faculty development can be targeted toward attitudes, knowledge, and skills for effective collaborative practice; capacity-building for self-assessment of team functionality; working together to determine the adoption of new information or policies and procedures; patient safety and quality improvement; leadership and organizational change; and general topics on teaching and learning (Silver and Leslie 2017). These authors go on to describe various teaching formats to consider, including case-based workshops, teambuilding exercises, peer coaching and mentoring, web-based learning, preceptorship training, longitudinal programs, communities of practice, and teaching tools and resources. Resources for faculty development in the effective delivery of IPE are provided by the IPEC through their Faculty Development Institutes (IPEC 2022). The previously mentioned IPEC core competencies (values and ethics; roles and responsibilities of collaborative practice; interprofessional communication; and teamwork and team-based care) form the foundation of their Institutes.

NAVIGATING GENERATIONAL DIFFERENCES IN IPE SETTINGS

Given the differences in demographics of health professions learners within and across disciplines, there is often broad generational representation among IPE learners. Where one health profession may have more senior students participate in IPE, another may introduce IPE to students very early in the curriculum. Additionally, the time required for completion of training differs widely across the health professions. The result is varying levels of maturity of learners in regard to both age and training. While this can provide a nice variety of perspectives that enhances the shared experience, it may also create challenges. Additionally, educators typically represent an older generation compared to learners, with a mix of Millennials, Gen X, and Baby Boomers, creating potential for contrasting expectations and attitudes toward teamwork, differing approaches to patient care, and varying styles of mentoring among IPE faculty/facilitators. The blending of generations across both IPE learners and educators necessitates a flexible approach to IPE to accommodate varying expectations and preferences, and consideration of the mix of generational representation among learners can enhance the effectiveness of the learning experience. In the following sections, specific guidance for delivery of IPE in health professions education across multiple generations in three key areas is provided: student engagement, effective use of student teams, and promotion of a relationship-rich learning environment.

Igniting and Maintaining Student Engagement in IPE

As with any educational program, learner engagement in IPE is key, making consideration of generational differences important to the development of effective learning opportunities. Being digital pioneers and digital natives, respectively, Millennial and Gen Z learners tend to be more technology-savvy and prefer learning activities that incorporate technology compared to older generations (Seemiller and Grace 2016). They may appreciate IPE that incorporates telehealth or simulation rather than group discussion in a classroom setting. When lectures are necessary to deliver foundational concepts in the didactic IPE setting, use of short, interactive videos may be more engaging than traditional classroom-based lectures. However, as stated in Chapter 5, instructors should use technology but know their limits regarding comfort level and proficiency with these tools.

Shortened attention spans and the need for immediate gratification have also necessitated a stronger emphasis on getting and keeping students' attention in the classroom. As discussed previously, lengthy lectures that promote passive learning are not readily embraced by newer generations of learners who crave more stimulation in the learning environment. Delivery of information in small bites via micro-lectures and the use of active learning strategies such as flipped classroom, audience polling, group cases, and problem- or team-based learning will result in greater student engagement and more effective learning, while still meeting the needs of older generations.

Best Practices for Multigenerational Teams

As mentioned previously, the four vital ingredients for effective performance of multigenerational teams are communication, inclusion, trust, and conflict resolution. IPE facilitators can support a shared understanding among team members of how the team will operate and resolve conflicts by providing necessary resources, including platforms for communication, tools for collaboration, and templates for team contracts. Facilitators can leverage technology to support teamwork, catering to the needs of Millennial and Gen Z learners. For example, learning management systems can be utilized for communication and shared document storage, as can texting, group chats, and collaborative tools such as Google Docs.

IPE facilitators should incorporate team building exercises at the beginning of the course to create a sense of belonging and cohesiveness among teammates. Exercises to help teammates get to know one another can create opportunities for learners to discover things they have in common with one another and to respect the personalities, backgrounds, and experiences that make them unique. As described in Chapter 5, inclusive teaching practices also support a sense of belonging and trust among team members and instructors. As stated previously, it is vital that all team members' voices are heard, and that each member has an opportunity to give and receive feedback from other team members.

Building and Supporting Relationships

Chapter 5 gives a lengthy description of the need for relationship-rich learning environments for Millennial and Gen Z learners. This is especially important for IPE due to diverse team member expertise and the need for mutual understanding and respect. IPE facilitators can support a relationship-rich learning environment by being easily accessible to students when they have questions or need immediate feedback. Likewise, peer mentoring among students in IPE teams can be an effective way to build relationships. A positive learning environment that promotes empathy for others and allows student choice is critical. Offering options and seeking student input on the learning approach support student agency. It is also critical to establish clearly defined expectations of students and teams at the beginning and throughout the course. Creating these relationships of mutual understanding and trust in both didactic and experiential IPE settings will ensure that the needs of Millennial and Gen Z learners are met.

CHAPTER SUMMARY AND CONCLUSION

While effective implementation of IPE presents its own challenges related to accommodating learners from diverse clinical backgrounds and professional cultures, the inclusion of learners and educators from various generational backgrounds creates further need for careful planning and attention to learner expectations. This chapter presented guidance for development and implementation of IPE programs in consideration of these differences.

Chapter 9 will further explore how the current generation of health professions students develops through experiential learning, particularly in their professionalism and professional identity formation, as well as through mentorship and role-modeling.

Chapter 9

Cultivating Professionalism and Professional Identity Formation through Experiential Learning

Health professions education is multifaceted, preparing the next generation of practitioners through didactic, experiential, and interprofessional learning experiences. The introduction of each new learning environment offers learners the opportunity to hone new skills and helps shape the type of practitioner they will be once they transition into practice. However, these learners are not truly exposed to or immersed in the professional roles and responsibilities expected of those entering the workforce until they embark on their experiential learning journey. This environment is often the first time these learners engage with practitioners working in the field and these experiences are crucial to ensure that the next generation are prepared for entry into practice upon completing their degree.

"Becoming a professional, exhibiting professionalism, and developing a professional identity are an interwoven, dynamic developmental process" (Moseley et al. 2021, 13). When considering Millennials and Generation Z learners, engaging with professionals in the field is crucial as they seek hands-on learning opportunities as they identify these experiences as creating the foundation needed for a successful career (Seemiller and Grace 2017a). This chapter examines experiential learning theory, as well as explores the role of professionalism in the health professions, how professionalism skills are cultivated throughout one's career, and how health professions education supports this cultivation through experiential learning. For the purposes of this chapter, professionalism is defined as an outward display of professional identity and professional identity is defined as an individual thinking, feeling, and acting as a professional in their field (Merton 1957; Moseley et al. 2021).

THEORY OF EXPERIENTIAL LEARNING

The theory of experiential learning proposes that learners acquire knowledge through transformational experiences. Seen as a holistic and adaptive learning process, experiential learning shapes learners through experiences, perception, cognition, and behaviors (McCarthy 2016). More specifically, "experiential learning is constructing knowledge and meaning from real-life experiences" (Yardley, Teunissen, and Dornan 2012, 161). This meaning is accomplished over four stages (concrete experience, reflective observation, abstract conceptualization, and active experimentation) and how a student navigates these four stages can be dependent on the subject or experience (Kolb, Boyatzis, and Mainemelis 2014; McCarthy 2016). Students also tend to favor one aspect of the cycle more than others, which often correlates to their preferred learning style, but to truly complete the transformational process, learners must go through all four stages.

Scholars have proposed that learning transfer does not carry over into practice if the learner does not have the number of situational cues needed to trigger the knowledge and skills required for real-world practice (McKeachie and Svinicki 2014). This discrepancy results in gaps in learning; however, when what is being learned matches the practice situation, transfer should be seamless. Hence the need for experiential learning. "If you want students to be able to transfer what they learn to the real world, it helps if the learning takes place under conditions that approximate the real world" (McKeachie and Svinicki 2014, 204). The integration of the real-world environment with real skills development and utilization should prepare learners for practice, as long as real problem-solving opportunities are embedded. Additionally, students should be reminded that experiential learning provides opportunities to learn about real-world practice and with a goal of learning, not just going through the motions (McKeachie and Svinicki 2014).

To create and implement experiential learning opportunities well, McKeachie and Svinicki (2014) outline key components that are essential to ensure that the intention of the learning experience is met. These include the following caveats: (1) the integration of real-world situations that students must address; (2) the inclusion of a complex and/or ill-defined problem with no easily identified answer; (3) utilization of tools available in the real-world setting; (4) the instructor should only serve as a resource and not guide the student through the task; and (5) once the solution is identified, the learner should actively reflect on the experience (to include their findings) and receive feedback on how they navigated the scenario. (McKeachie and Svinicki 2014)

While the inclusion of experiential learning is important, identifying appropriate strategies for assessing these experiences is also critical. The integration of this learning approach supports student learning assessment related to collaboration, communication skills, leadership, and professionalism (Bradberry and De Maio 2019). The "concrete" nature of experiences places the learner within a real-world setting, ensuring that students see the ramifications associated with decision making, clinical practice, and so forth. Students are no longer protected from seeing both the positive and negative outcomes that can result from practice.

Medical education applies the principles of experiential learning to experiences that place learners in clinical settings with practicing professionals to establish an authentic learning environment (Yardley, Teunissen, and Dornan 2012). These experiences prepare learners to think, act, and feel like a practitioner, further shaping their professional identity while also enhancing their professionalism through interactions with their clinical preceptor. A deeper and more intentional look at professional identity formation and professionalism will be explored later in this chapter.

Some medical education scholars pose that to provide students with a robust clinical experience, educators must also consider how social learning theory applies to the learning experience. "Social learning theory is a theoretical perspective on how experience and its learning consequences are essentially located in social milieus" (Yardley, Teunissen, and Dornan 2012, 162). Essentially, theorists believe that the learner influences the learning environment, and the learning environment influences the learner. This multidirectional impact clearly aligns with professional identity formation and professional development, as each of these fundamental concepts acknowledges that individuals change over time due to their own personal experiences and the environments in which they navigate. Moreover, with each new experience, the learner must reflect and adapt to how it affected them and recognize that previous experiences will shape how they approach their next one. Furthermore, they must also recognize that they will continue to be reshaped with each new experience and will continue to do so throughout their lifetime.

While most health professions refer to experiential learning using this vernacular, medical education also refers to it as workplace learning (Yardley, Teunissen, and Dornan 2012). Yardley, Teunissen, and Dornan (2012) note that workplace learning should be disbursed and occur throughout the curriculum, and not only toward the end. This early learning helps to shape and reshape how students will learn once they enter their clerkship experiences and residency rotations. Action research examining these types of learning experiences have identified common themes which include learner importance, acceptance within the workforce, situational understanding and workplace integration, and active and meaningful participation in workplace functions (Yardley, Teunissen, and Dornan 2012). It is essential to ensure these experiences are not superficial if educators expect learners to engage, and instilling linkages between experiences will enrich learning further.

Students engaging in workplace learning are "seeking to construct a sense of identity as well as gain knowledge and skills and will therefore appreciate any help you can give them to relate experiences to their personal career goals" (Yardley, Teunissen, and Dornan 2012, 163). Workplace responsibilities should increase over time to promote learners' feelings of commitment and belonging to the organization and profession. Learners who fail to connect to their workplace will feel excluded which will negatively impact learning.

Within nursing education, experiential learning is critical as there are fewer opportunities for students to learn within the hospital setting (Grace et al. 2017). Active engagement is required for experiential learning and educators should strive to cultivate within learners the behaviors and attitudes needed to provide quality patient care. This cultivation should occur across the curriculum and should be designed to build clinical competence prior to practice while also fostering person-centered skills.

PROFESSIONALISM AND PROFESSIONAL IDENTITY FORMATION

Professionalism has long been an area of discussion within the health professions as each discipline struggles with voicing what professionalism truly means within their field (Birden et al. 2014; Cruess, Cruess, and Steinert 2016; Fitzgerald 2020; Holden et al. 2015). Each health profession has their own set of values, attitudes, and behaviors that influence how professionalism is developed within future generations of health professionals (Ford and Moseley 2020; Jha et al. 2015). The dynamic nature of health professions education, with its immersive experiences and clinical skill development, has created a false sense of self-driven professionalism within its learners. Historically, educators have used the "see and do" approach to learning to instill the basic principles of professional practice, failing to recognize that mentorship is essential to ensure that students are identifying the unique characteristics and traits needed for the practicing professional. This trend is apparent in medical education and has been further exacerbated by the complexity of distinguishing between professionalism and professional identity formation. Yet, these limitations are not only found within medical education; other health professions also struggle to integrate professionalism into their existing curricula (Mylrea, Gupta, and Glass 2015). A concept analysis by Fitzgerald (2020) set out to examine how other health professions scholars defined professional identity and professionalism, and initial analysis found that many scholars used terms such as professionalism, professional self-concept, and professional socialization synonymously. Overall, Fitzgerald found that professional identity definitions varied greatly when an explicit definition was provided. However, prior to delving into the differences between the two, let us first examine Chickering and Reisser's (1993) theory of learner development and the correlation of vectors that establish identity, cultivate purpose, and develop integrity and how these vectors impact the role of professionalism and professional identity formation within the health professions.

Chickering and Reisser's Learner Development Vectors

As two of the leading seminal theorists in learning theory, Chickering and Reisser (1993) proposed a view of student development theory that deviated from the existing literature and supports the fluctuating nature of student progression within higher education. While this theory was first noted in the early 1990s, its relevance remains today, especially as it speaks to the holistic development of learners. Both Millennial and Gen Z learners look for those experiences that will further define who they are as individuals and as future practitioners. Chickering and Reisser's student development theory articulates this critical developmental process, and it aligns well with the expectations of these two generations of learners' expectations. Devised into seven vectors (developing competence, managing emotions, moving through autonomy toward interdependence, developing mature interpersonal relationships, establishing identity, developing purpose, and developing integrity), Chickering and Reisser (1993) proposed that learners rarely fit within one pathway, that movement along that path may vary between learners and within the same learner, and that movement between vectors may occur separately or at the same time. For the purposes of this chapter, the authors identified the interconnectedness between establishing identity, developing purpose, and developing integrity to how learners nurture professionalism and professional identity formation throughout their academic programs and beyond.

The first key vector for examination is establishing identity. Identity development is "the process of discovering with what kinds of experience, at what levels of intensity and frequency, we resonate in satisfying, in safe, or in self-destructive fashion" (Chickering and Reisser 1993, 42). The elements of establishing identity support acceptance of one's body, appearance, gender, sexual orientation, and sense of self. The authors expound on the elements of sense of self by examining this evolution within the context of social, historical, and cultural caveats. Furthermore, they examine how it is impacted by one's role, lifestyle, reaction to feedback, acceptance, and self-esteem.

Furthermore, Chickering and Reisser note that this development is tied to one's stability and integration into society. When considering generational cohorts, Millennials have been viewed as a very accepting generation. However, Gen Zs have surpassed Millennials in their inclusion of diversity and individuality (Shatto and Erwin 2016; Wilkins 2021), embracing the fluidity of gender identity and failing to see the need for categorization of oneself (Seemiller and Grace 2019a).

Developing purpose is the next vector within the model and examines one's ability to assess interests and options, to clarify goals, to make plans, and to persist despite obstacles. These plans contain three fundamental elements: vocational plans and aspirations, personal interests, and interpersonal and family commitments. At this stage, an individual must be able to evaluate how one's lifestyle, family, and profession impact future goals, and should drive the learner's decision-making process.

The final vector within this structure is developing integrity. While closely related to establishing identity and developing purpose, this stage tasks the learner with establishing the foundation needed to interpret experiences, guide behaviors, and maintain self-respect. Three overlapping stages occur during this development and include humanizing values (transitioning from uncompromising belief systems to principled thinking), personalizing values (affirming one's core values and beliefs while respecting others' differences) and developing congruence (matching personal values with socially responsible behaviors).

These three vectors speak to an individual's ability to recognize their own sense of self, their identify within the confines of their professional aspirations, and how these aspirations shape their sense of purpose. While the theorists did not specifically include the role of professional identity formation and professionalism within these vectors, the correlation of these developmental elements within health professions students is clear. The alignment of the vectors and experiential learning are fortuitous as learners enter these final developmental stages during a pivotal period of learning where students are being exposed to and learning from those active practitioners in the field. The convergence of learning, mentoring, and student development sets the stage for a student to evolve and grow, forming their personal and professional identities before adopting the values that will drive how they engage with others throughout their lifetime. (Chickering and Reisser 1993)

Millennials and Generation Z Views of Professionalism

Millennials and Gen Zs have similar and differing expectations of the workplace. For Millennials, many view their careers as opportunities to "finance their personal lives, including travel, expensive electronics, and trendy clothes" (Seemiller and Grace 2016, 5). They also have high expectations regarding pay, advancement, and work-life balance. While money is a driver for this generation, they are more likely to remain in a work environment that pays less if it hosts a strong culture, offers work-life balance, provides resources needed for job optimization and skills development, and opportunities for growth (Phillips 2019). Millennials' connections to their friends and family have challenged how many view the traditional workplace, with many utilizing working hours to remain engaged with those outside contacts, blurring the lines between work and personal life.

As more Gen Zs enter the workforce, many will push to alter or eliminate the traditional expectations associated with the professional world. Gen Zs strive to remain connected and engaged with others so the likelihood of them working a traditional 8 to 5 workday is minimal (Seemiller and Grace 2016). They will seek out professional opportunities that provide optimal flexibility. This flexibility and connectedness also extend to their workplace environment to include consideration of whether working in a traditional office space is needed. All these factors will impact how they view professionalism.

Millennials and Gen Zs do see eye to eye when seeking out work that they view as fulfilling. Both generations strive to identify a career that allows them to pursue what they identify as meaningful. Both generations view their professional lives as opportunities to fill a need either within the organization or the world. This compulsion to leave their mark will impact how they approach work and what drives them to remain engaged.

Professional Identity Formation

"Professional identify formation, or PIF, represents the transformative process of a lay person into a professional" (Moseley et al. 2021, 11). Shaped by an individual's experiences and those they are exposed to within the professional setting (Mylrea, Gupta, and Glass 2019), PIF challenges learners to think, act and feel like a practitioner within their respective fields (Moseley et al. 2021; Dall'Alba 2009). While there is some disagreement as to the timeframe during which professional identify formation occurs, scholars agree that this process primarily transpires during formal education and practice (Mylrea, Gupta, and Glass 2015). PIF is unique to each individual and is impacted by the context and environment to which the learner is exposed. Authentic experiences are more likely to impact PIF, and the inclusion of experiential learning opportunities within the practice setting further shape this identity development. Furthermore, this formation pushes learners beyond just knowledge and skills, striving to foster the development of a holistic learner that can critically apply what they learned into practice and continue to grow as a practitioner.

The inclusion of PIF within health professions education is a growing need (Mylrea, Gupta, and Glass 2017) and should be a welcome inclusion for both Millennial and Gen Z learners. Since the turn of the century, PIF "has been recognized as an essential aspect" within most health professions disciplines to include dentistry, medicine, nursing, and pharmacy (Cruess, Cruess, and Steinert 2016; Mylrea, Gupta, and Glass 2017). Yet, while many have identified a need for increasing the presence of PIF in health professions education, there is a lack of understanding of what PIF means and how it should be aligned within the existing curriculum (Mylrea, Gupta, and Glass 2017; Trede, Macklin, and Bridges 2012).

The integration of authentic learning experiences is an expectation of both generations, as each strive to have a stronger understanding of what will be expected when they enter the workforce. Gen Zs, in particular, prefer to observe and practice (Shatto and Erwin 2017), which aligns with the increased popularity of YouTube. The inclusion of experiential learning within health professions education fills a critical need and ensures that learners are exposed to real-world application and practicing professionals.

As a result of the protective nature of their parents, as previously discussed in Chapter 5, many Gen Z students may need further development in their professionalism skills and as a result need additional support with the formation of their professional identity (Wilkins 2021). Educators may encounter students who have never been employed or only held temporary or short-term jobs. This lack of employment may have led to minimal engagement with active practitioners in their prospective career fields or a lack of preparation when it comes to identifying potential preceptors or mentors when entering their internship or clinical rotations.

The role of PIF within health professions education is still evolving as educators struggle to distinguish the differences between professionalism and professional identity formation. Universally, "all health professions are guided by a set of values, attitudes, and behaviors" (Ford and Moseley 2020, 200) that help to establish and cultivate professionalism within the profession (Jha et al. 2015). The interconnectedness and complexity of professional identity formation and professionalism creates challenges when developing learning experiences as each strives to produce a well-rounded and well-prepared practitioner while also having differing outcomes that each rely on the other to achieve this goal.

PROFESSIONALISM IN THE HEALTH PROFESSIONS

Historically, professionalism has not been taught formally with the curriculum, but development in this area has been expected (Cruess, Cruess, and

Steinert 2016). Over the last several decades, there has been a focused examination of what professionalism means, behavioral expectations, strategies for teaching professionalism, and lastly, how it should be assessed. Yet, while additional attention has been placed on addressing these goals, no universal interpretation of professionalism has been identified (Mylrea, Gupta, and Glass 2015; Trede, Macklin, and Bridges 2012). This lack of a consistent definition may be the result of educators interweaving professionalism and PIF.

Within medical education, many educators overlap these two developmental roles. Cruess, Cruess, and Steinert (2016) proposed that teaching professionalism correlates to a student's professional identity development, and that evaluating a learner's development in this area will show progression within professionalism. Others stipulate that PIF, and experiential learning are required for professionalism to occur (Mylrea, Gupta, and Glass 2015). Like professional identity formation, professionalism develops over time, hence why this development is directly linked or overlaps with professional identity formation.

Concerns regarding the lack of professionalism within health professions students is significant as this often leads to issues of misconduct or fraud (Mylrea, Gupta, and Glass 2015). The literature also contrasts what is a core value of the profession and what is practice (Regehr 2020). Regehr (2020) comments on how the evolving nature of society has influenced the core values and practice expectations of health professions. For example, in his commentary, he discusses the changes to professional dress and whether it is truly a practice expectation or a value of the profession. He discusses that at one time neck ties were seen as the epitome of professionalism for male health practitioners but now to reduce risk of infection, they should be eliminated. While this change is directly correlated to a practice change, it also shows correlation with value changes of the profession as many practitioners recognize the need to be seen as more relatable by patients in order to provide the best possible care.

Many educators may struggle to teach their students professionalism as they are tasked with teaching not only the core values and practice expectations of the profession, but as they will also be expected to share their own individual core values to instill an authentic relationship. In recent years there has been discussion of the potential negative outcomes related to professionalism within the clinical environment. As students enter into practice settings, they may be exposed to practitioners who may not represent the ideals of the affiliated academic program or who may fail to represent the profession positively simply due to their own personal experiences (Lockwood, Jordan, and Kunda 2002). The inclusion of professionalism early in the curriculum should bolster students' abilities to identify those traits that do not align with the direction of the profession and those that do.

Professionalism and Medical Education

Medical education has long struggled with defining professionalism as a discipline. This led to the Liaison Committee of Medical Education (LCME) revising accreditation requirements in the early 21st century to include professionalism as a competency (Cruess et al. 2014; Moseley et al. 2021). While many medical educators agree that professionalism is a key component of medical education curricula, they fail to understand how to successfully prepare learners for entry into the profession. Desy, Reed, and Wolanskyj note that questions regarding professionalism of Millennial learners began with "the enforcement of work-hour restrictions in medical education" (2017, 247). Many practicing physicians felt that these learners viewed their work as shift work and that work-hour restrictions impacted continuity of care and patient interactions. Additional concerns stemmed from a lack of personal boundaries specifically tied to their use of social media and the associated risks this use could have on breaches of professionalism and protected information.

Professionalism in Nursing Education

The role of professionalism in nursing education is interwoven within the formation of professional identity. Professionalism is the ninth domain within the 2021 *Essentials* and is described as the "formation and cultivation of a sustainable nursing identity, accountability, perspective, collaborative disposition, and comportment that reflects nursing's characteristics and values" (American Association of Colleges of Nursing [AACN] 2021, 11). The overlapping nature of PIF and professionalism is not surprising, as many scholars have argued that the duality of these two areas are challenging to separate and define. The AACN expands upon their definition to state that professionalism "encompasses the values of integrity, altruism, inclusivity, compassion, courage, humility, advocacy, caring, autonomy, humanity, and social justice" (AACN 2021, 49). It is a nonlinear and continuous process that requires ongoing engagement upon entry into practice by supporting the development of others in roles such as educators or preceptors as well as in a mentorship. Professionalism continues to grow and change with every challenge and experience and matures with each passing year.

Professionalism in Pharmacy Education

In 2000, pharmacy educators reemphasized the critical role professionalism held within pharmacy education, specifically noting it as a critical component within education and practice (Boyle et al. 2007). A white paper developed by the American Pharmacists Association (APhA) Academy of Student Pharmacists (ASP)/American Association of Colleges of Pharmacy (AACP) Council of Deans (COD) Task Force "identified several issues involving professionalism and described specific strategies to enhance professionalism within pharmacy education and the early years of pharmacy practice" (2000, 1). The white paper strived to define professionalism not only for student pharmacists but practicing pharmacists as well. In 2011, a revised list was published and included 11 specific traits: (1) knowledge and skills; (2) a commitment to self-improvement and lifelong learning; (3) a service minded orientation; (4) pride in the profession and dedication to advance its societal value; (5) covenantal relationship with those served; (6) alertness, creativity, initiative and innovation; (7) conscientiousness, integrity, and trustworthiness; (8) flexibility and punctuality; (9) performance accountability; (10) ethically sound decision making and moral behaviors; and (11) leadership (Mylrea, Gupta, and Glass 2015).

NAVIGATING PROFESSIONAL IDENTITY FORMATION IN HEALTH PROFESSIONS EDUCATION

Distinguishing professional identity formation and professionalism development is a long-standing issue within health professions education as many educators struggle with identifying how to evaluate this development across the curriculum (Cruess, Cruess, and Steinert 2016; Cruess, Cruess, and Steinert 2019). Formed by internal and external factors, PIF requires social interaction and for the learner to evaluate both how they see themselves and how others see them (Noble, McKauge, and Clavarino 2019).

Taylor and Harding (2007) stipulate that PIF is an element of undergraduate education, but it is important to recognize that PIF is ongoing and must continue to be cultivated following entry into practice. This development is supported through positive role modeling and mentoring, timely feedback, and self-driven reflection. This holistic approach ensures that learners and later practitioners are consistently evaluating how internal and external factors shape their professional views.

As previously discussed in Chapter 6, within medical education, Miller's Pyramid of Assessment has long been thought of as the exemplar for evaluating student progression within clinical skill development (Miller 1990). Miller's model purposes four assessment levels: knowledge, competence, performance, and action. The proposed integration of clinical skills assessment prior to rotations allowed educators to evaluate clinical skills performance prior to entering the healthcare facility for rotations. Furthermore, this allowed true clinical encounters to meet the needs for high-level, individualized assessments and objective structured clinical examinations (OSCEs) to serve as preparatory assessments that did not directly impact patient care.

In recent years, Cruess, Cruess, and Steinert (2016) proposed an amendment to this model to add identity as a key element. Transitioning Miller's Pyramid from four tiers to five, the authors proposed the addition of the "is" element at the top of the model to allow educators to assess students as they transition into their clinical experiences (Cruess, Cruess, and Steinert 2016). The "is" addition focuses on a learner's ability to "think, act, and feel" like the practitioner they have trained to become (Cruess, Cruess and Steinert 2016, 181). The integration of authentic learning experiences is essential to foster professional identity formation and these experiences are further enhanced when integrated into the practice setting. The addition of this layer adds complexity to the model but highlights the important role this formation has in shaping future healthcare practitioners.

Within pharmacy education, educators recognized the need for further examination of professional identity formation and its impact on student pharmacist development. To address this gap, the AACP developed a task force dedicated to examining the role of PIF and how it should be assessed. The 2019–2020 AACP Student Affairs Standing Committee was charged with investigating the role of PIF as a transformational practice model. Within its report, the standing committee noted that professional identity change "goes beyond acquiring knowledge ('thinking') and displaying professionalism ('acting') to include the pharmacist's perceptions of self ('feeling')" (Welch et al. 2020, 1402). The committee also identified five strategic goals that the AACP organization should adopt to promote PIF advancement within pharmacy education. These goals included developing a PIF framework; creating a PIF culture within pharmacy education, training, and practice; establishing teaching and facilitating best practices for PIF; faculty and preceptor development to adopt and address PIF in curricular, co-curricular, and extracurricular activities; and establishing assessment best practices for PIF (Welch et al. 2020). Due to the timeliness of this report, limited findings are available as to how this call to action has impacted PIF within pharmacy education and more time is needed to see how pharmacy educators will address this need.

Mentoring

The origin of mentoring was first seen in Homer's *The Odyssey* where Mentor was responsible for educating Odysseus's son Telemachus while he was away fighting in the Trojan War (Odell 1990). The relationship between Mentor and Telemachus was not limited to solely relaying knowledge and skills but was instead comprehensive, extending to all aspects of the pupil's life. A key factor of this relationship dynamic was the intentional feedback Mentor provided regarding errors Telemachus made, which supported his continued development and growth. Mentor established the fundamental aspects of the mentoring dynamic, which requires the educator to be "intentional, nurturing, insightful, and supportive" (Odell 1990, 6).

As history has shown, mentoring should be an active and engaging process that occurs frequently. This dynamic relationship should not be limited to just classroom experiences but should extend outside the traditional curriculum to include discussions regarding career advancement, professionalism, professional identity, and research (Evans and Forbes 2012). To create an authentic mentoring relationship, both faculty and students must be prepared to be open and honest for relationship building to occur. Listening is critical for faculty, specifically during discussions related to the student's future goals and aspirations.

The evolving landscape of higher education places an increasing need for strong mentoring relationships and positive role models. These dynamic faculty-student relationships support students as they transition from learner to practitioner. The mentoring dynamic is considered a relational process, which allows faculty to transfer knowledge, wisdom, experience, and so forth to the mentee at a critical time to promote development (Evans and Forbes 2012). Furthermore, these relationships allow students to emulate the characteristics and behaviors they hope to adopt upon joining the workforce, thus enhancing their professional identity formation and professionalism (Mylrea, Gupta, and Glass 2015).

How a student's professional identity is shaped is greatly influenced by role models and mentors (Cruess, Cruess, and Steinert 2019; Wilkins 2021). Millennials and Gen Zs seek out mentoring relationships and see it as an important aspect of professional development. Both generations expect these relationships to provide structure and guidance to support their continued development (Desy, Reed, and Wolanskyj 2017; Eckleberry-Hunt, Lick, and Hunt 2018; Ford and Moseley 2020; Swanzen 2018;). Millennials prefer one-on-one mentoring that aligns with their individualized learning plan (Desy, Reed, and Wolanskyj 2017; Evans and Forbes 2012). These individualized experiences allow them to thrive and support their preference for a structured academic environment. They also look to these collaborative relationships as mechanisms to aid professional growth and continued development.

Gen Zs place value on their relationships with mentors, with many seeking these connections to better prepare for entry into practice (Seemiller and Grace 2019; Wilkins 2021). They look for mentors who are accessible and will look to their mentors to set the boundaries of the relationship (Eckleberry-Hunt, Lick, and Hunt 2018). It is important to note that while mentees expect to be exposed to high quality mentor modeling, if they cannot identify with the faculty member, they will withdraw from the relationship (Weinberg 2019). Therefore, relationship building is critical to the mentoring dynamic as was previously discussed in more detail in Chapter 5.

While mentees may be fearful of vocalizing their deficits to their mentors, they will strive to impress them as they want their mentors to value their contributions to the relationship and see them as a partner. Yet, to successfully engage with their mentors, Gen Zs need clearly defined expectations supported with individualized feedback delivered in a timely manner (Eckleberry-Hunt, Lick, and Hunt 2018; Ford and Moseley 2020; Swanzen 2018). Educators should not assume that subtle feedback will be effective with this cohort (Eckleberry-Hunt, Lick, and Hunt 2018) and should strive to have an authentic relationship with full transparency (Seemiller and Grace 2017b).

Evans and Forbes (2012) found that mentoring health professions students should include four elements: digital literacy, immediate connectivity, experiential, and things that matter. Mentors should focus on digital literacy as the internet and technology have changed how students access information to include availability of information that would have not been easily on hand in the past. Faculty will need to guide learners through this information to ensure that they know how to navigate through useful and extraneous information. A focus on immediate connectivity is also important as mentors must set boundaries within the mentor-mentee relationship. "Today's mentee demands more time and attention than in years past because of the assumption of instant access" (Evans and Forbes 2012, 400). Both Millennials' and Gen Zs' views on boundaries differ from previous generations and they will need clearly defined expectations at the initiation of the mentoring relationship regarding how and when to communicate.

As mentees expect to be connected, they will also want to have real-world experiences. This expectation of experiential learning will task the mentor with guiding students as they take their first steps into the professional world. This guidance may include helping foster professionalism or professional identity as well as helping students navigate initiating research or developing presentations and/or manuscripts. Lastly, mentors should be prepared to help their mentees with things that matter to them and be aware that the mentor's research agenda may not be the same as students.' Both Millennials and Gen Z learners want to engage in projects that impact others and mentors may need to help these students understand how their interests impact the world around them (Evans and Forbes 2012).

Overall, it is essential to identify the type of mentorship the student is looking for as not everyone will expect the same level of interaction. The link between mentoring and professional identity formation is clear as "work and identity reinforce one another and that role modeling will interact with these processes to produce learning outcomes" (Weinberg 2019, 427). Also, it will be crucial to assess the level of mentorship needed for the learner to help them achieve their goals and be prepared for entry into practice. Lastly, providing timely evaluations and feedback is critical to ensure that progression is occurring.

Mentoring Relationships in the Clinical Setting

As educators, it is important to recognize that students' mentoring experiences vary based on the learning environment. Health professions students spend significant time within the clinical skills environment, which poses additional challenges outside of traditional learning to include increased anxiety and burnout (Jordan et al. 2019). This will be examined shortly. Tuomikoski et al. (2020) found that to develop clinical competence within nursing students requires a learner to engage with clinical practice nurses and that these relationships are critical to support and enhance learners' clinical knowledge and skills. Bhatnagar et al. (2020) also found that mentorship in medical education has been shown to improve clerkship grades, increase match rate, and improve residency applications. "During the clinical practice period, the student gains practical competence, is taught how to link theory into practice, becomes familiar with the social culture of the profession, learns how to work in and lead a team, and becomes adept at organizing overall nursing care" (Tuomikoski et al. 2020, 2). Positive mentorship in the clinical environment should lead to student competence if a trusting faculty-student mentoring relationship is established. Furthermore, these relationships also influence a health professions student's overall feeling regarding their profession.

Yet, while the mentoring relationship focuses primarily on the faculty-student relationship, it is not uncommon for clinical mentors to feel that they are not prepared to support students within these relationships. Many clinical mentors may seek out opportunities to enhance their own clinical skills and look to their institutions to provide developmental support (Tuomikoski et al. 2020). This skill development will often focus on developing learning objectives, strategies for giving and receiving student feedback, and mechanisms for integrating technology into the clinical environment.

Clinical mentors should also be cognizant of rotation-related stressors and develop strategies to support their students as they complete their clinical experiences. "Lowering anxiety is important because students who are highly anxious may be less successful academically, suffer detrimental physical and mental health effects, and may be unable to interact effectively with patients or team members" (Cornine 2020, 231). Student anxiety can be reduced when they engage with faculty who display caring attitudes and utilize humor and other positive teaching behaviors. These positive relationships have also been shown to reduce burnout (Jordan et al. 2019). Bhatnagar et al. stress that "[w]ithout the appropriate availability of mentorship, medical students eager for this resource may be at a disadvantage in terms of preparation for residency applications, professional development, and discovering an interest in an academic career" (2020, 8). While this statement is specific to medical education, its transferability to other health professions is apparent. Health professions clinical faculty must be prepared to support not only the academic pursuits of their students but to also support their mental and physical health as well.

Role Modeling in Health Professions Education

Desy, Reed, and Wolanskyj (2017) note that Millennials want structure, direction, and to understand expectations that are essential aspects of the mentorship dynamic. Furthermore, they seek one-on-one mentorship that allows their learning to be authentic and customized to their needs. Essentially, they prefer experiential learning to gain hands-on experience guided by their mentors, as this provides them with an authentic learning environment in which to hone their clinical skills (Desy, Reed, and Wolanskyj 2017). This learning environment pushes clinician educators to have dual roles—that of mentor and role model. While the symmetry of these dual roles is clear, it also speaks to the influence these educators have on steering the future of the profession as they set the expectations and goals for the next generation of practitioners.

A key aspect of successful mentoring "involves mentee emulation of a model mentor's behaviors" (Weinburg 2019, 428). To accomplish this goal, role modeling is essential to provide a student with a model in which to emulate. By asking the student to mirror practitioners' behaviors, the student should begin to feel more comfortable within the clinical environment and when engaging with patients. The integration of student-driven discussions and patient interactions will also provide educators the opportunity to identify how their role modeling has influenced the student's professionalism and professional identity formation over time and provide feedback when needed.

Within their early research, Seemiller and Grace (2016) found that Gen Zs had clear expectations regarding those individuals that they viewed as role models. Their positive parental relationships greatly influenced what they viewed as important within the mentoring relationship. As Gen Zs had open and honest relationships with their parents, they will seek out these same attributes within their mentors. This research also showed that along with their K–12 teachers, Gen Zs tended to recognize sport coaches as role models/mentors because they used positive reinforcement and communication skills to motivate them and engaged them within the decision-making process so that they felt included and heard (Seemiller and Grace 2016). These findings are key as they speak to how educators should approach role modeling and that this generation would be open and willing to see faculty as someone who could fill this role. The integration of positive communication strategies while also providing specific and firm expectations should result in positive role modeling sessions.

EXPERIENTIAL LEARNING WITHIN HEALTH PROFESSIONS EDUCATION

Historically, students display passive learner tendencies, acquiring knowledge through the traditional learning environment. Yet, research continues to find that active learning strategies, to include experiential learning, result in increased retention and improved critical thinking skills (Bradberry and De Maio 2019). The inclusion of experiential learning is crucial as it provides an opportunity for learners to "engage in professional and productive learning activities," which allows students to construct knowledge while being able to "actively engage with and critically reflect" on what they are learning (Bradberry and De Maio 2019, 94, 95). Furthermore, students who participate in experiential learning are more likely to apply the knowledge, skills, and values they have acquired to real-world situations, which should result in producing career-ready graduates (Fewster-Thuente and Batteson 2018).

Bradberry and De Maio note that as educators "we want our students to develop critical thinking abilities, written and oral communication skills, and the capability to research and analyze" (2019, 95). The acquisition of these skills supports student success upon entry into practice and their ability to utilize knowledge they obtain in the learning environment within a real-world setting. Furthermore, they are then able to take this existing knowledge and construct new knowledge and connections between both existing and new knowledge to navigate these novel experiences thus resulting in deep learning. The development of these problem-solving and critical thinking skills will be critical as health professions students become health professionals.

Due to the hands-on nature of the healthcare environment, health professions education has long embraced the role of experiential learning opportunities within their curriculum (Grace et al. 2017). While the role of experiential learning varies across health professions education, most health professions programs utilize these learning opportunities to prepare learners for future practice. The integration of these learning experiences helps to shape learners' understanding of practice and to identify the qualities and behaviors they strive to have upon entry into the profession. The following sections will address how experiential learning is evaluated and how it impacts professional development.

Role of Experiential Learning and Professionalism Development

Both Millennials and Gen Zs gravitate to learning experiences that have a direct link to their future career, often seeking out those experiences that offer hands-on learning and practice (Hampton and Keys 2016; Seemiller and Grace 2019a; Wilkins 2021). As previously discussed, Gen Zs, in particular, seek out practice experiences that allow them to connect with and learn from mentors. These connections are key as they allow the learner to observe and practice, which aligns with their preferred learning style (Chicca and Shellenbarger 2018; Shatto and Erwin 2016; Wilkins 2021).

Experiential learning affords the perfect opportunity for students to experience the clinical world prior to becoming a practitioner. Clinical rotations and clinical experiences serve as ideal mechanisms for exposing learners to positive and sometimes inadvertently negative role models, which should result in a learner cultivating their professionalism and professional identity. These hands-on experiences often result in a student identifying how they want others to view them as professionals and allows them to enter the workforce better prepared for the challenges that lay ahead.

Transitioning from Experiential Learning into the Workplace

As both Millennials and Gen Zs enter the workforce, they often lack or have limited work experience. As a result, these generations will need strong mentoring relationships to ease the transition (Wilkins 2021). As Gen Zs navigate the work force, it will be imperative for them to identify workplace mentors as they will want to forge new connections. Wilkins notes that "a generation that has experienced continued support and been taught to fear failure will benefit by the engagement of mentors who genuinely care about their success" (2021, 33). While Wilkins was primarily focusing on Gen Z learners and their faculty mentors, this sentiment is very applicable to the work environment. Generally, Gen Zs often lack professionalism skills, even following entry into the profession. This development will be ongoing as well as the continued formation of their professional identity. They will require feedback and guidance as they navigate their professional lives to foster their decision-making abilities and to help bolster their confidence (Chicca and Shellenbarger 2018; Wilkins 2021).

Many Gen Zs view their relationships with their supervisor as transactional (Seemiller and Grace 2016). While this generation appreciates organizational hierarchy, they do not always view those in leadership as being mentors. As such, providing the necessary mentorship to foster continued professional development may be challenging.

"Millennials straddle the line between respecting authority and feeling that leadership is out of touch" (Phillips 2019, 15). This generation is very sensitive to leadership dynamics, noting when attention is paid primarily to others and not to them. This failure to acknowledge their worth and contributions will result in them feeling ignored. The consequences of this slight will result in decreased productivity over time and a lack of allegiance to the organization (Phillips 2019).

Additionally, Millennials tend to turn away from leaders who promise the world and fail to deliver on those promises. This lack of follow-through often impacts Millennial workers' productivity, which will decrease each time they are faced with a failed promise (Phillips 2019). By including Millennials within the organizational process, they will gain a sense of satisfaction and are more likely to remain engaged and committed to their job. Retention of trained employees benefits employers by reducing the cost of turnover and recruitment.

The overarching work environment will greatly influence Gen Zs as they navigate their professional careers. They will view a less-structured organizational culture as inviting as it will allow them to work more effectively. Furthermore, they will gravitate to employment opportunities that offer flexible scheduling, project-based work, and self-defined work hours as they seek versatility within their workday to achieve personal and professional goals (Seemiller and Grace 2016). If they are unable to find this type of environment, they are likely to seek employment elsewhere or simply create the job they want on their own.

CHAPTER SUMMARY AND CONCLUSION

Experiential learning challenges students to grow personally and professionally by exposing them to practitioners in their field. These experiences further shape their professional identity and professionalism through mentoring and role modeling. The intentionality of experiential learning pushes learners to enhance their knowledge and skills, allowing them to move beyond what they originally learned in the classroom and ensuring over time that their sense of purpose and legitimacy within their professions continues (Yardley, Teunissen, and Dornan 2012).

The penultimate chapter of the book examines the value of a college degree in the labor market to include a health professions degree as well as the projected return on investment of a college education. Chapter 10 also examines perceptions of worker preparedness, and employer satisfaction with college graduates. Furthermore, this chapter investigates the impact of COVID-19 on the healthcare workforce, and how Millennials and Generation Z navigates the workplace.

Chapter 10

Generational Differences in the Health Professions Workforce

Each generation brings to the table a different set of skills, expectations, and culture which must be successfully navigated. Intergenerational mingling does not always occur which has the potential to negatively impact worker productivity (Gerhardt, Nachemson-Ekwall, and Fogel 2021). It will be important for employees and employers alike to integrate strategies to work effectively as a team. When addressed, productivity can be increased.

Whereas ten or so years ago Millennials were the youngest generation in the workforce, this is no longer the case. Gen Zs have begun their foray into the professional world, which has resulted in substantial changes. This generation has grown up in a time of self-employment and as a result may be less inclined to work for others (Seemiller and Grace 2016). This is an important factor for educators to consider as these learners may seek to gain better basic skills while pursuing their college degree, and as they are fiscally driven, they may seek to shorten their collegiate time by enrolling in additional classes to allow them to enter the job market more quickly (Seemiller and Grace 2017b). It will be important for institutions to identify strategies or pathways for non-business majors to enroll in coursework.

When considering the health professions, there are additional layers of complexity that are added, specifically related to interprofessional teams, quality patient care, and effective patient and team communication. As healthcare practitioners spanning multiple generations learn to perform together in an evolving workforce environment, there are many concerns to be addressed including how to welcome Generation Z practitioners, how to supervise across generational divides, and how to navigate the complex post-COVID labor market landscape. It will be necessary for healthcare practitioners to continue to evaluate the added value of college degrees. Employers will need to examine how to retain workers who are satisfied, well-trained, and engaged. Employees must strive to collaborate in experiential learning environments, pushing past differences and appreciating how unique generational traits can yield shared values. This chapter explores the impact multigenerational employees have within the labor market, specifically the healthcare industry, and how Millennials and Gen Zs have impacted the healthcare field as a profession.

DEMONSTRATING THE VALUE OF A COLLEGE DEGREE IN THE LABOR MARKET

Throughout most of the 20th century, the college degree was considered a benchmark to achieve to ensure one would have a successful career (Wingard 2022). Many employers have used this designation as a basic requirement for certain types of jobs. This resulted in a reciprocal relationship or understanding among colleges and employers, where institutions of higher learning produced something that industries wanted and needed. Degree seekers and employers saw the college degree as a credential demonstrating value, which often led to the acquisition of stable jobs with opportunity for growth, and in turn, the prospect of a life of financial security for college degree holders. Additionally, this label of being college-educated often led to status within the community and to the perception that a person had the ability to be a leader, to serve in community organizations, or to give advice personally and professionally.

A report by the American Association of American Colleges and Universities (AAC&U) found that of the 496 employers surveyed, 63% held "quite a lot" to "great deal" of confidence in higher education in 2018. This increased to 67% in 2020 (Finley 2021). When asked if getting a college degree was worth it, 42% said "it definitely" was in 2018 and increased to 49% in 2020. Yet, while the findings were positive overall, when the data was broken down by employer age, there were distinct differences. When considering whether a college education was worth it, 54% of employers 40 years of age or under said "it definitely" was. However, only 39% of employers 50 years of age or older said it was worth it. These findings also varied based on educational background; of those with postgraduate degrees, 59% said it was definitely worth it as compared to those with a bachelor's degree (47%) and those with an associate degree or less (28%). (Finley 2021)

Even when the COVID-19 pandemic arrived in 2020, college graduates experienced lower rates of job loss compared to high school graduates. In many cases, college graduates were able to work from home while bringing in their same salary, while fewer workers with a high school diploma reported the ability to do their work remotely (Wingard 2022). Nonetheless, Wingard (2022) predicted that this value is shifting, and that students and employers will seek more flexible and affordable methods to achieve the same ends. In health professions education, however, a certain level of specified training is certainly required. The consideration of how a college degree is valued is a complex question that can vary among the perspectives of each worker, each employer, and across varying fields of study and practice.

The Value of a Health Professions Degree

In a *US News and World Report* article titled "Are Medical School and Becoming a Doctor Worth It" (Kowarski 2020), several interviewed physicians commented with responses that fell somewhere in a range of "it depends." For many of the physicians, medicine was a "calling," and the abilities and autonomy that they possess in helping people are unparalleled. However, several also noted that medicine should not be something practiced just to make money; in this case, they felt, it would not be worth the trouble. There are many professions that provide the opportunity to earn a high income. Practicing medicine, while certainly in this category, comes with a great deal of personal, financial, and time sacrifices to get to the end goal. The interviewed physicians also mentioned the frustrations of dealing with the commercialization of healthcare, insurance companies, and other administrative burdens that can impair one's ability to enjoy the satisfaction of working in a helping professions role (Kowarski 2020). Certainly, across the healthcare professions there are unique considerations to take into account as one determines whether it is worth it when thinking of pursuing education and entering the workforce within a particular area of study and practice.

For instance, while there are certainly careers that pay higher than nursing, many who have entered the profession have found a positive return on investment (Carlson, 2023). In 2021, registered nurses earned a median salary of approximately $77,000 annually, while nurse practitioners earned approximately $118,000 annually on average. These salaries are competitive with other fields in and out of the medical professions in respect to salary and duration of education; for example, also in 2021, physician assistants earned a median annual salary of $121,000. Further, a career in nursing can lead to lifelong careers, flexibility in employment choices, and the benefit of a fast-paced and ever-changing work environment (Carlson, 2023). Practitioners of other medical professions are weighing in as well. The year 2023 marked seven straight years of dentistry listed as a *US News and World Report* "100 Best Jobs" profession (American Dental Education Association, 2023). Additionally, projections show that employment in dentistry will increase by 7.6% (over 10,000 new dentist jobs) by 2028.

College Graduates Falling Short in Preparedness for Work

Beyond a student/practitioner's personal perception of worth when it comes to their credentials, degree attainment, and the practice of their profession, other constituents are weighing in on this question of worth as well. Employers and institutions of higher learning are also invested in determining the value added to the workforce from degree attainment.

An AAC&U employer study (Finley 2021) found that employers saw room for improvement regarding college graduates' preparation for work and that there was variability between graduates. When survey participants were asked how satisfied they were with college graduates' abilities with skills application and the knowledge they acquired to manage complex problems in the workforce, 49% of employers indicated they were very satisfied. Employer satisfaction differed by age with 59% of employers 40 years of age and younger indicating they were very satisfied as compared to 28% of employers 50 years of age and older. The employers with postgraduate education (57%) were more satisfied than employers with a bachelors (47%) and an associate degree or lower (35%) (Finley 2021).

According to a study by Wingard (2022), college graduates across the board were struggling to apply what they learned in the classroom to real-world experiences. Also, employers reported that current college graduates were lacking critical thinking, writing, and oral communication skills, compared to several years prior. Interestingly though, college students still believe that they are signing up for the same value and the same credential that will bring about steady employment. What is causing this discrepancy in the perceived value and the employer perception that is occurring for many graduates?

Wingard (2022) comments that employers perceived that colleges were not always keeping up with changing needs. For example, changes in technology, products, services, and the skills needed to manage in today's market have resulted in a need for curricular change. If employers do not feel like they are getting their return on investment (ROI) from new graduates, soon college graduates will feel the same. Wingard (2022) suggested that the ROI from a college degree peaked around 2010 and that within the next few decades there will be new paths for gaining the credentials and skills needed by employers.

THE GREAT RESIGNATION AND RELATED WORKFORCE TRENDS

As colleges and higher education practitioners are concerned with helping students to develop skills that will prepare them for careers, those who work in colleges and universities will likely find themselves perplexed when the labor market fluctuates or demonstrates unusual patterns. While employers have strong assertions about workers preparedness, employees, on the other hand are reaping the benefits of a labor market that has trended to their advantage, offering more than enough job choices for those looking for work, or looking to change their work (Feldmann 2022; Pizzinelli and Shibata 2022). In spring 2022, Pew Research Center released a post exploring the reasons that workers cited for leaving jobs in 2021 (Parker and Horowitz 2022). The authors stated that the massive job losses experienced by workers earlier in the pandemic set off a chain of events that led to the Great Resignation in 2021. As of November 2021, the US "quit rate" was at its highest point in two decades. Results from the Pew Research Center survey revealed employees' top ten reasons for leaving a job in 2021, from highest to lowest, as follows: low pay; lacking opportunity for advancement; feeling disrespected in the workplace; childcare; lack of flexibility; poor benefits; need to relocate geographically; feeling overworked; working too few hours; and unwilling to receive a COVID-19 vaccine. A separate survey question asked broadly whether the respondent's reason for leaving their job was related to the COVID-19 pandemic, and 31% responded yes (Parker and Horowitz 2022).

The survey indicated that of those who quit a job in 2021, 78% are now employed (Parker and Horowitz 2022). A majority of these respondents claim that it was "easy" to find their current job. Additionally, most of the re-employed respondents view their new jobs as an improvement, citing factors such as more money, better upward trajectory, better work–life balance, and more flexibility. Of course, responses vary by demographics, and there are still notable numbers of workers who are less happy or see no improvement with their new employment. However, the overall trends suggest that workers saw an opportunity to take advantage of a market that had swung in the direction of their favor, seizing the opportunity to search for greener pastures. (Parker and Horowitz 2022)

Telehealth and Flexibility

Seemiller and Grace (2016) projected that Generation Z employees would value flexibility in regard to how and when they are able to complete their work. In recent years, many Gen Z and Millennial students experienced a time of necessary flexibility during the remote learning phase of the COVID-19 pandemic. It is interesting to consider how dispositions toward flexibility or experiences in being allowed flexible modalities might impact workers' demands going forward. As workers in varying fields of practice search for new opportunities with better pay, work–life balance, and flexibility, how might healthcare professions keep up?

For example, Beetham, Fiellin, and Busch (2022) found that many physicians used telehealth for the first time during the COVID-19 pandemic. Telehealth allows flexibility for both patient and provider regarding receipt and provision of care respectively. Twenty-nine percent of surveyed respondents indicated using telehealth prior to COVID-19, a rate that increased to 66% to include those who had used telehealth after the start of the pandemic. The majority of respondents found telehealth to be more effective than they would have expected. An even larger majority supported the idea of telehealth flexibility becoming permanent after the pandemic (Beetham, Fiellin, and Busch 2022).

During the spread of the pandemic, telehealth became a viable way to conduct nonessential appointments. Routine visits could take place in a setting that allowed both the patient and physician to be at home. This was useful for patients but also for physicians who may have been quarantined themselves (Hyder and Razzack 2020). The authors noted that for telehealth to be a success, providers and patients must be on board. The authors also stated that socioeconomic and generational factors among patients can affect their acceptance of telehealth options. Digital natives, or those less than 35 years old, were surprisingly found to be less trusting of telehealth reliability, as compared to older generations who had simply adopted a preference for digital options. Those outside of health professions were generally less likely to have knowledge related to telehealth, but those with a college degree in any field were more likely to be proficient in using telehealth compared to those without a college degree. The authors concluded that education around telehealth will be crucial for its acceptance, and this includes Generation Z patients (Hyder and Razzack 2020). Whether flexibility is offered to healthcare practitioners through telehealth or other means, it will be crucial to address worker preferences in certain healthcare professions in which there are not enough workers to meet demand.

Worker Shortages in Some Healthcare Fields

Overall, there is predicted to be an increasing shortage in the number of healthcare workers compared to demand, occurring within the next few years (Duquesne University School of Nursing 2022; Zhang et al. 2020). Estimates show that a deficit of 18 million healthcare professionals will occur by 2030, and that over half of this shortage will be in the nursing profession (Mao et al. 2021). This shortage in healthcare professionals has been a long time coming.

> According to the Health Resources and Services Administration's (HRSA) report in 2011, there were an estimated existing deficiency of 17,722 primary care providers in the United States of America. Furthermore, in 2020, the United States of America may face shortages of 45,400 primary care physicians and 46,100 medical specialists—a total shortage of 91,500 doctors in 2020 (Zhang et al. 2020).

While these shortage predictions focused primarily on medicine and nursing, these shortages extend to other health-related professions as well.

There are several reasons for this projected shortage. In part, it will be due to the number of individuals in the aging Baby Boomer population who will require greater and more frequent care in the coming years (Flaherty and Bartels 2019). As medical advances occur, people live longer, which means more chronic conditions, and more people who are needing care for an extended period of time, as compared to previous generations. Flaherty and Bartels (2019) note that over the next decade of the 69 million older adults living in the United States, that two-thirds will be managing multiple chronic conditions.

As the population of individuals over 65 years of age should nearly double in the next decade, this trend will also mean the retirement of current working physicians included in this demographic (Caplan 2023; Duquesne University School of Nursing 2022; Flaherty and Bartels 2019). Further, as many practicing physicians are choosing to enter specialties, it is projected that there will be a drastic shortage of those in primary care or family medicine. Shortages will likely also occur in other healthcare fields. Projections show that the demand for nurses possessing a bachelor of science in nursing (BSN) will increase at a greater rate than the supply over the next five years (Duquesne University School of Nursing 2022).

While many have recognized the impending healthcare worker shortage for quite some time, this shortage has been further exacerbated by the COVID-19 pandemic. A study conducted by Novilla et al. (2023) found that those frontline healthcare professionals working during the pandemic reported increased stress (97%), anxiety (86%), and exhaustion and burnout (76%). While the healthcare system is still navigating the impact COVID-19 had on its healthcare workforce, the potential long-term ramifications are present (Assistant Secretary for Planning and Evaluation 2022).

Solving this problem will require enrollment increases and recruitment efforts for healthcare education programs. However, schools may face a challenge in doing so due to increasing shortages in healthcare faculty, particularly nursing. Some nursing programs have reported turning away qualified applicants due to not having enough faculty members (Aragon et al. 2020; Duquesne University School of Nursing 2022; Rosseter 2022).

Cooper (2022) discussed the state of the nursing shortage in 2022. As fewer individuals choose to pursue nursing and existing practicing nurses leave the industry, hospitals are losing money. In order to maintain staffing, hospitals must pay exponentially more to employ travel nurses as well as increase their financial output to retain and recruit permanent staff through higher salaries and large sign-on bonuses. Nonetheless, the nursing shortage is only expected to increase into the 2030s (Cooper 2022; University of St. Augustine for Health Sciences 2022).

While many healthcare professions are experiencing worker shortages, others have demonstrated potentially opposite outcomes. Lebovitz and Rudolph (2020) discussed projections that the number of PharmD (doctor of pharmacy) graduates will outpace the demand for pharmacist jobs. The authors commented that the number of pharmacy graduates and the perspectives of schools graduating new pharmacists do not match the job landscape. Instead, the authors suggested training pharmacy graduates who can market their skills to a variety of related jobs. The job market issue could also be corrected by reducing class sizes or reducing the number of PharmD programs. Additionally, as prospective students become aware of this shift in supply and demand, they may choose not to study pharmacy. Either way, the authors discuss that pharmacy schools will need to accept that their graduates may no longer be predominately employed at chain and community dispensing pharmacies. Helping students and employers to recognize the value of a PharmD education beyond these roles could be a positive strategy, as there are many careers that require a graduate level science background (Lebovitz and Rudolph 2020).

Projecting worker shortages within healthcare fields is challenging as it is hard to predict future needs as compared to health professions enrollment. While following the COVID-19 pandemic, most health professions programs experienced decreased enrollments, this trend could be altered should a world changing event occur in the coming years. This is a dynamic and evolving process that requires constant monitoring to truly determine the future of the health professions workforce.

MILLENNIALS IN THE WORKPLACE

As discussed earlier in this chapter, hosting multiple generations in the workplace can be challenging and can result in friction between the generations (Delgado et al. 2020; Gerhardt, Nachemson-Ekwall, and Fogel 2021). This is especially true as each generation may foster different expectations regarding work–life balance, recognition, and feedback. Navigating these multigenerational workplaces will require employers to recognize and adapt to the conflicting expectations of these differing generations.

By 2025, Millennials will comprise three fourths of the workforce (Brant and Castro 2019) and expect high rewards for the work they do (Delgado et al. 2020). "[M]illennials find a significant importance in bonuses, pay, and prefer having leaders that take care of them on the basis of individuality" (Delgado et al. 2020). They thrive in constantly evolving environments due to their ability to adapt quickly, and their early exposure to technology makes them adept at multitasking between devices.

However, there is a growing body of literature that labels this generation as entitled (Brant and Castro 2019). There is some debate regarding the validity of this stereotype with some arguing that this generation's actions are due in part to the environment in which they grew up (Brant and Castro 2019). They came of age during the time of the Great Recession and as a result they had limited job prospects when they entered the job market. They often struggled to find employment, or they took positions in which they were overqualified (Brant and Castro 2019). "Average incomes of millennials fell at twice the rate and have recovered at a much slower pace compared with those of older generations" (Brant and Castro 2019, 529). This has resulted in this generation being faced with increased debt and a higher cost of living.

When considering the healthcare workforce specifically, Millennials comprise almost half of current healthcare workers (Bittner 2019). Yet, healthcare organizations are struggling to retain Millennials, especially in the nursing field. The rationale behind their departures is unclear; although, this lack of retention is often tied to the need for additional leadership training (Delgado et al. 2020; Bittner 2019). Implementing intentional mentorship programs should foster retention by creating an environment in which Millennials thrive. These mentorship programs should create a system of support as well as provide a consistent feedback loop to allow these employees to develop, grow, and address their mistakes (Delgado et al. 2020; Bittner 2019).

GEN Z IN THE WORKPLACE

In the last four to five years, the first Generation Z individuals began graduating from college, entering the workforce, attending graduate school and/or professional programs, and entering specialized professions, including jobs in healthcare settings (EAB 2018; Pew Research Center 2019). As these digital natives with memories of growing up in the Great Recession enter professional settings, differences among them and prior generations of workers, including their immediate Millennial predecessors have become apparent. They expect real-time communication and responses, more frequently utilizing tools like messenger applications or Slack. They expect video content to be incorporated into recruitment, professional development, and normal working communications. They can be less collaborative than Millennials, in that they may prioritize their individual success over team success in a work setting. However, they are competitive workers, and tapping into their desire to win can promote a collaborative and driven environment (EAB, 2018).

Gen Z Workplace Preferences

Seemiller and Grace (2016) predicted that Generation Z individuals, as employees, would be less tied to the traditional 8 o'clock to 5 o'clock workday. As this generation is accustomed to connectivity at all hours of the day, they may desire to complete their work on their own terms and desire flexible working arrangements, in regard to the time and space in which their work is completed (Seemiller and Grace 2016). Seemiller and Grace (2017b) found that nearly 50% of Gen Zs want to work for themselves, which will create challenges for employers as more of the older generations retire. They also noted that Gen Z workers will likely be impacted by observing the "creative entrepreneurship" models of companies such as Airbnb, Craigslist, and Uber (Seemiller and Grace 2016). Through such services, workers can set their own terms to an extent, without having to own a business. The secondary income that these opportunities provide for some has generated a greater value in autonomy related to how one works. Seemiller and Grace (2016) also predicted that Gen Z individuals would prioritize engaging in work that is both meaningful and leads to change for the greater good. They may do this by finding a way to turn their passion into paid work.

Frahm (2019) noted that acknowledging Generation Z expectations can be crucial in bridging workplace generational gaps. In general, Generation Z workers expect flexibility, respect from their mentors, an opportunity to make a difference, frequent feedback, and space to create new ideas. Frahm described the Gen Z need for flexibility as promoting a "work-life blend" as opposed to the traditional work–life balance (2019, para 19).

Seemiller and Grace (2016) discussed how to relate to Gen Z, using strategies that can be helpful to college teachers and administrators, but also to employers anticipating their arrival within workplaces. The authors emphasize that it is important to find the best strategies for relating to Gen Z as people. Interestingly, despite their comfort and ease with connecting virtually, many Gen Z individuals value opportunities to communicate face-to-face. Additionally, Gen Z are realistic, and they value transparency. Gen Z will consult their parents on many decisions, even as they are entering adulthood;

therefore, forming a connection with Gen Z individuals may involve connecting with—or at the least, respecting their bond with—their families (Seemiller and Grace 2016).

Also important is the environment in which Gen Z students/employees work. They will prefer an environment that protects their physical safety, as well as an environment that feels inclusive and supports their mental health and holistic well-being. For workplace environments that involve learning from a mentor, Gen Z appreciates being consulted and part of the learning process, rather than being taught at. They also appreciate learning from peers. It is also important to remember that this generation does appreciate collaboration, but often on their own terms after an opportunity for independent work. Additionally, Gen Z appreciates technology incorporated into their learning, and they value experiential learning. They also like training opportunities that are connected to real-life scenarios and will prioritize working toward goals that are clearly connected to values (Seemiller and Grace 2016).

MULTIPLE GENERATIONS PRESENT IN THE WORKPLACE

When multiple generations are present in the workplace, their values may be different, in addition to differences in how they communicate, how they solve problems, how they build relationships, and how they lead. This can cause conflict, or alternatively, workplace leaders can see an opportunity to promote supportive behaviors among the generations present. For example, generally tech savvy younger generations, such as Millennials and Gen Z, could intimidate less technically inclined generations with their quick technical literacy and skill, or they can support others who are less well versed in these areas in a collaborative manner. Health organizations should focus on promoting professional socialization and feelings of workplace citizenship among its employees, across generational divides (Srinivasan 2012).

Differences across generations in the workplace affect how people interact along five key variables, according to Srinivasan, "work and life related values and motivators; professional growth; attitudes to rules, authority, and hierarchy; attitudes to learning, training, and development; and work environment" (2012, 55).

Bridging the Gap among Generations in the Workplace

To lead Generation Z individuals in the workplace, it can be helpful to understand what makes them unique—culturally, socially, from a motivational standpoint, related to technology, and in how they communicate. In addition to exploring what sets younger generations apart, workplace leaders should also explore what generations have in common. The older generations in today's workforce may have started working young and plan to retire later. As a result, as Generation Z enters professional realms, there are four to five generations present. Each generation has experienced entering the workforce under its own unique set of obstacles. As such, they have different views of how they value work and how they balance it with other aspects of their lives. Further, how each generation displays professionalism may vary (Frahm 2019).

Frahm (2019) suggested that to understand any generation and how its members navigate the workforce, five factors should be considered: economic factors, political happenings, social change, technological advances, and landmark events. Just as importantly as navigating these differences in generational background, Frahm (2019) emphasized the importance of considering how the current workplace generations are similar. The author suggested that likely all workers had similar dreams and goals when starting their careers (e.g., ambition, a desire for upward mobility, and a need to seek feedback from colleagues and mentors). Frahm (2019) identified fairness, growth, and community as workplace values that all workers strive to obtain, no matter their generational traits.

Mentoring across Generations in the Workplace

Frahm (2019) recommended that older workplace generations embrace that their role as a mentor matters to Generation Z. Those leading Gen Z employees can improve workplace dynamics by encouraging brief communication, going digital, and incorporating social media. Additionally, workplace training can be structured to provide regular feedback, positions can be crafted with clear operational goals, and individual contributions can be mapped to organizational goals, all strategies that help Gen Z see the "why." Frahm (2019) also suggested that leaders take caution not to equate generational traits and character flaws as synonymous. It can be far too easy to stereotype other generations in such a diverse workplace. In reality, many issues with coworkers are due to situational factors that could be problematic coming from any generational standpoint. There are quality workers with high standards across all generations; keeping an open mind is how these individuals should work together (Frahm 2019).

Understanding worldview and motivational factors can be important for supervisors who are managing across generations in the workplace. Having grown up in the recession, Gen Zs are quite aware that hard work and intelligence are only part of what it takes to get and maintain a good job. This generation is entering the workforce acquainted with the realities that jobs are partially about survival, and given an economic turn, they could become even harder to find (Seemiller and Grace 2016).

CHAPTER SUMMARY AND CONCLUSION

Many changes have transpired in the workforce since the onset of the COVID-19 pandemic, some challenging, some inconvenient, and some unexpected but overdue (Feldmann 2022). Employees are eager to explore options that meet their needs as workers, professionals, and individuals. As such, many companies are attracting new employees, who are eager for a change, with competitive salary packages; however, in some fields, tenured workers' salaries are lagging, contributing further to the continuation of the Great Resignation. Further, workers realized that they could perform adequately under flexible work conditions during the height of the pandemic, and they continue to demand this flexibility in addition to other perks (Feldmann 2022).

To keep pace with an evolving job market, employers will need to pay close attention to what employees need and want, from a recruitment and retention perspective, particularly in health professions facing shortages. Additionally, in health professions fields facing a surplus of new professionals, the idea of finding the right "match" will be key (Lebovitz and Rudolph 2020; Pizzinelli and Shibata 2022). It is crucial to help graduates explore how their knowledge and skills are transferable, while considering the unique generational trends that are also contributing to labor market changes. Ensuring that health professions employees are in a work setting which they find rewarding and meaningful is no one-size-fits-all task. Creating work environments that are safe, collaborative, and productive will require a balance between strategic individualization and a careful focus on shared values among cross-generational professionals.

The final chapter brings us full circle and summaries best practices for teaching and learning across the generations. Chapter 11 summarizes findings and sets the stage for the upcoming generation, Generation Alpha.

Chapter 11

Best Practices for Navigating the Generational Divides

Previous chapters have outlined the similarities and differences between the newest generation to enter higher education, Gen Zs, and Millennials in the context of an evolving higher education landscape and how these factors influence learning preferences, skill development, co-curricular experiences, and team dynamics. This chapter focuses on a discussion of the trends affecting higher education in general and health professions education, specifically, their impact on the workforce, and the role of interprofessional education (IPE) to support team readiness. The chapter concludes with best practices for education to apply for Gen Z and Millennial learners and a brief introduction to Generation Alpha.

PROJECTION OF HIGHER EDUCATION MOVING FORWARD

At the time of publication of this book, as higher education institutions make their way out of a global pandemic and continue to navigate new economic and demographic realities, taking an honest look at the current landscape is imperative. Institutions are anticipating a "demographic cliff" (Grawe 2018, 45) that will come to fruition in the late 2020s, due primarily to a decline in the number of upcoming high school graduates, which will result in fewer college applicants (Brown 2022). With fewer potential students to enroll, institutions will need to focus on retention, just as heavily as recruitment (The Chronicle of Higher Education 2022). Additionally, as the traditional enrollment funnel has been compromised (Povejsil 2021) and certain demographics of students are enrolling at lower rates, institutions will need to consider non-traditional populations of prospects and strategies for recruiting these learners (e.g., adult learners).

While a college degree has been considered a benchmark achievement toward obtaining a desirable career for some time, Wingard (2022) predicted that in the coming decades, the idea that college equals gainful employment will no longer be a given. Of course, in healthcare fields, the need for credentialed professional training will persist. However, remaining competitive in an evolving higher education market may prove to be a challenge for institutions and programs. Graduate and professional programs must consider what employers desire and the jobs that are vacant, as they guide students in refining their knowledge, skills, and abilities into professional interests (Lebovitz and Rudolph 2020). For health professions students, this meaning-making can occur in part through experiential learning and immersive experiences (Yardley, Teunissen, and Dornan 2012).

In line with the idea of experiential learning settings, going forward, it will be important to remind educators that learning occurs within many contexts, in and out of the classroom. The ways in which students remain engaged (with each other, with their institutions, and with their fields of study) and the ways in which they develop as holistic individuals are not "extra" components of the learning environment, but rather, vital ones. For this reason, student affairs/student services work is referred to as "co-curricular," indicating that spaces outside of the classroom are a necessary part of the educational experience (Roberts 2019). Further, the many ways in which students stay engaged and constantly connected are vital components of how they uniquely develop as a generation of learners.

EVOLUTION OF HEALTH PROFESSIONS EDUCATION AND LASTING IMPACT ON THE WORKFORCE

A 2021 report by IBM estimates that, by the year 2025, there will be over 38.6 billion smart devices connecting us to one another and generating huge amounts of data (Jackson, Lin, and Sávio 2021). As of April 2022, an estimated 5 billion people use the internet and 4.65 billion use social media (Statista 2022). All of this "connectedness" will have a profound impact on the evolution of health professions education as innovative technologies enter the classroom. Such growth is vital to keep pace with the desires and expectations of Millennial and Gen Z learners.

Healthcare has seen the rise of immersive technology, such as augmented reality (AR) and virtual reality (VR), for both learning and skill development (learner-facing) and direct patient care (patient-facing). These technologies provide opportunities for learning in low-stakes, safe environments, as well as the ability to connect to and interact with others without regard to geography. Price points for AR and VR devices continue to drop while technological advances keep developers on their toes. This translates to wider accessibility to these technologies by demographic groups who previously could not afford them and improved access by educational institutions.

Other examples of technology use in the classroom to engage learners include internet-based audience-response systems, podcasts, social media, poverty simulation games, artificial intelligence (AI)-driven communication training programs in VR or AR, and casting of smart devices to monitors so that students can work collaboratively on a project. The latter is a common element of active learning classrooms that have been incorporated into facilities that house health professions education programs. Both Millennials and Gen Z learners value real-time feedback, which can be supported through the use of technologies such as video conferencing and video- and audio-enabled grading systems. The increasing rate of acceleration of technological advancements in education, coupled with the propensity for these generations to embrace these technologies, will have a lasting impact on the workforce by shaping applicants' expectations of their future work environments. Even so, advancement of technologies like VR and artificial intelligence can introduce real problems in the classroom. For example, AI can be used to create written products, introducing issues of academic dishonesty that are incredibly difficult to detect (Broadsky 2022; Peritz 2022). As these technologies continue to advance at lightning pace, educators and employers will need to be vigilant—ready to reap the benefits while avoiding the negative impacts.

The inclusion of immersive technologies aligns with the new curricular structures health professions programs are adopting. The incorporation of competency-based education (CBE) is becoming more widespread as it prepares learners for entry into practice. CBE is an evidence-based approach to teaching and learning that allows students to progress through training programs at their own pace, so long as they are able to demonstrate certain competencies as identified through backward curricular design. In true CBE, progress is not time-bound, making this challenging for programs that are lockstep in nature to accommodate this approach. Elimination of grades is a transition that may prove difficult in regard to faculty buy-in. Health professions programs are turning to more competency-based or competency-driven curricula to align with the training needed to develop a practice-ready graduate, but true alignment is not always possible.

Despite the growing popularity of CBE, faculty often face challenges in its implementation. Such challenges include discomfort with previously established cut points for progression and hesitancy to hold students back when they fail to reach these thresholds. There may be a need to revisit cut points if many students fail to succeed yet approaches for revising these are not always clear. Development of timely and responsive remediation plans may also prove challenging, inhibiting successful implementation of CBE.

As discussed in previous chapters, Millennials and Gen Z learners appreciate direct expectations that align with learning. However, these generations have rarely experienced failure so supporting them when they fail may be difficult. Learner development in the context of helicopter and co-pilot parents often creates an expectation among learners for mentoring alongside the curriculum. As discussed in Chapter 9, the need for additional mentoring can add complexity to the implementation of CBE.

One potential approach to improve alignment between CBE and actual practice is for the learning environment to support deep learning. Branzetti and colleagues (2019) describe deep learning as taking what is learned and constructing knowledge, with a drive for self-directed learning beyond the classroom. While foundational knowledge is critical in health professions education, taking learning a step forward through critical thinking and application to building upon prior knowledge can close the gap between curricula and actual practice. Learning how to learn becomes a critical element to prepare learners to succeed in an evolving workforce and to grow as practitioners (Fink 2013). Deep learning may resonate with Gen Zs, who tend to be self-directed in their learning (Seemiller and Grace 2016).

In the current learning and workforce environment, skill development becomes a critical part of health professions education. A focus on clinical skills training can provide hands-on experience that prepares learners for a competitive workforce. Development of these skills may also help learners successfully immerse themselves into the learning environment on their experiential rotations, providing a more authentic learning experience, which Millennial and Gen Z learners highly value. "Power skills," formerly described as "soft skills" are increasingly critical in the development of a practice-ready graduate of the health professions. These skills include leadership, communication, conflict resolution, critical thinking, decision making, empathy, giving and receiving feedback, resilience, and teamwork (Flanagan 2022). Gen Z learners will need to differentiate themselves from other applicants by demonstrating mastery of these skills, given the current landscape of a competitive job market. Gen Zs, who highly value professional development and lifelong learning, are more likely to embrace opportunities for reskilling and upskilling, and in an increasingly fast-paced world, businesses are apt to view a culture of continuous learning as a competitive advantage (Perna 2021).

Role of Interprofessional Education (IPE) to Foster Professional Development and Team Readiness

Navigating the complex nature of healthcare requires health professions education to prepare learners for the dynamic and varied nature of the profession.

To achieve this goal, the integration of IPE, professionalism, professional identity formation, and continued lifelong learning must be embedded to foster success as learners transition into practitioners. While IPE is not a new concept, many health professions educators continue to struggle to successfully integrate these experiences into their existing curricula. Challenges such as access, time, support (both faculty and institutional), and resources serve as roadblocks and can lead to negative or inadequate experiences for students. It is critical that each institution evaluate how IPE aligns with their overall learning goals so a comprehensive plan can be created. The implementation of a university-wide initiative or center is key to ensure that individual academic programs have the resources and support needed to effectively integrate these experiences; furthermore, a centralized initiative will allow the institution to utilize fiscal resources strategically and reduce redundancy across the institution.

Embracing the importance of professionalism and professional identity formation (PIF) within the curriculum is vital to promote positive learner development. The diverse nature of health professions education requires educators to prepare learners to adopt and embrace the values, attitudes, and behaviors of the discipline (Ford and Moseley 2020; Jha et al. 2015). Traditional health professions education has used the "see and do" approach to instill principles associated with professional practice but has struggled to strategically integrate and evaluate professionalism and professional identity formation within the curriculum. However, in recent years, professional identity formation has become a key aspect of health professions education with many recognizing it as an essential aspect of the profession. The integration of authentic learning experiences, clinical skills development, and intentional mentoring will foster a learner's sense of professionalism and professional identity. The adoption of these types of experiences will push learners to move beyond what they learned in the classroom and shape how their knowledge and skills will be used within professional practice.

OVERARCHING BEST PRACTICES FROM EDUCATION TO PRACTICE

"Teaching effectiveness will likely increase with careful examination of [Gen Z] attributes among health professions students, as well as the feasibility of introducing curriculum change within the context of health professions education" (Attardi et al. 2021, 2). Adapting to the needs of learners is a vital component of the teaching and learning environment, especially when navigating the expectations of multiple generations. The following sections provide overarching best practices for supporting learners as they transition from student to practitioner.

Curricular Development Strategies for Millennials and Generation Z

Considering how each generation processes information is important and can result in more strategically designed experiences. For example, Gen Z students prefer more clearly articulated instructions or guidance documents (Greico 2020). These learners are drawn to documents that allow the learner to easily discern the intent of the assignment and can see how each piece aligns with the other. While many faculty may view this as a simple component to incorporate, it can set the stage for a positive learning experience and ease the student's transition into the course or experience.

Millennials and Generation Z learners thrive within a learning environment that supports the incorporation of active, practice-based learning as they need to see how what they are learning will be incorporated into real-world practice. For educators, this means the incorporation of theoretical frameworks that support this learning approach and identifying theorists or scholars that recognize the utility of creating a faculty and learner supported environment. An example of this strategy is presented through L. Dee Fink's Taxonomy of Significant Learning, which focuses not only on strategies for supporting student learning but also provides approaches for introducing, preparing, and supporting faculty as they integrate this framework into their coursework. This taxonomy outlines six essential elements: foundational knowledge, application, integration, human dimension, caring, and learning how to learn (Fink 2013). Fink recognized that higher education had to move beyond Bloom's Taxonomy to create meaningful and intentional learning experiences. Designed to focus on the role of change within learning, Fink encourages educators to integrate significant learning experiences that will create lasting change, with each element of the taxonomy providing a distinctive value for the learner. Fink's taxonomy strives to foster a learning environment of constant change, pushing both educators and learners to examine how real-world practice demands academia to constantly update and elevate what is being taught in the classroom.

Strategies for Student Engagement

While curricular development is certainly at the heart of the educational experience, engaging students from a co-curricular standpoint is a necessary part of their development as well. If students are to have a well-rounded college experience, they must be meaningfully engaged in and out of the classroom

(Roberts 2019). The concept of student engagement from a co-curricular perspective is particularly important in "helping professions" such as student affairs and certain healthcare education fields (Perez 2016). As health professions students are learning how to help others through their future career, it is crucial that they receive the care and services they need to remain engaged in an environment that fosters their development. A learning environment that provides both psychological and physical safety is necessary to properly support students (Mundell 2022). An important aspect of providing this sense of safety involves coordinating services that help students in prioritizing their mental and physical health, in addition to their sense of belonging (Chidiac et al. 2018; Gopalan, Linden-Carmichael, and Lanza 2022; Pfeifer et al. 2022). Additionally, intentional mentorship opportunities can play a large role in how students develop into professionals and can increase the likelihood that the student/future practitioner will remain engaged throughout their career, in research and clinical pursuits (Hirsch et al. 2014).

With the propensity for these generations to embrace, even expect, use of technology in the classroom, incorporating various technologies can be useful to engage Millennial and Gen Z students. However, the choice to use technology should be guided by feasibility and the utility that it adds to the learning experience, rather than just the novelty of the technology. In other words, adding tech for the sake of adding tech is not practical or effective. But adding it to increase engagement and enhance learning can be beneficial. Though typically used in the K–12 environment, the SAMR (Substitution, Augmentation, Modification, and Redefinition) model is a useful framework for selecting, using, evaluating, and integrating technology in the college classroom (Hamilton, Rosenberg, and Akcaoglu 2016; Puentedura 2014).

The first two rungs on the ladder represent enhancement of learning through digital technologies. Substitution is replacing traditional materials and activities with digital ones, without any other changes to content. Augmentation involves incorporating digital enhancements, like hyperlinks, multimedia, or gamification, without changing content. An example would be incorporating digital portfolios to showcase work. The last two rungs on the ladder represent transformation of learning through novel approaches. Modification involves significant redesign and may be accomplished by larger changes, such as adopting a learning management system to connect students to manage the logistics of the learning experience. And lastly, redefinition involves creating new activities that fundamentally transform the classroom. Examples include blogging, podcasting, and virtual field trips. Professional development in the use of these technologies will become critical to stay abreast of the latest innovations and for skill-building in successful implementation approaches.

As discussed in Chapter 3, shifts are expected in demographics and enrollment of students in institutions of higher education in the coming decade. With these shifts, institutions will need to be responsive to the needs of Gen Z and Millennial students, as well as non-traditional students. Straddling these generational divides could prove challenging for educators. An in-depth understanding of the needs and expectations of these learners will be critical. Chapter 5 discusses in great detail these expectations and how they will shape higher education in the near future.

The needs of future learners will include robust support for mental health and accommodations for disabilities, as mentioned in Chapter 4. It is likely that, as consumers, students will seek out these services and base their application and enrollment decisions upon the variety and accessibility of such services at their prospective institution. Therefore, institutions will need to invest financial and human resources into building and maintaining these services.

Also discussed in Chapters 3 and 4, online learning, though much more widespread in the years during and following the COVID-19 pandemic, will be an even more important consideration for the next generation of learners who value use of technology to improve accessibility and practicality of information delivery. Virtual communities, such as those supported by platforms like GroupMe, have grown in popularity with the influx of Gen Z learners in higher education, who value connectedness and immediate feedback, especially via technology. These platforms are often preferred over email and text as a means of communication by Gen Zs. Even so, they do tend to prefer in-person interactions for social aspects and feelings of connectedness.

As mentioned in Chapter 9, Gen Zs and Millennials tend to pursue efforts that they perceive as meaningful and those that make them feel as if they are fulfilling a critical need. Accordingly, engagement will be greatest if they see a clear purpose to learning activities and perceive them to be beneficial to their future careers. This may be why learners from these generations tend to enjoy and value experiential learning, which provides them with hands-on experiences that are very relevant to the work they plan to do after graduation.

CONTINUOUS PROFESSIONAL DEVELOPMENT FOR FACULTY/EDUCATORS

Utilization of Centers for Teaching and Learning

Just like students, educators are expected to grow and learn, and continue to develop professionally. This is true on many fronts, including how to effectively teach to and interact with the student body. As mentioned elsewhere in this book, it is important for educators to have an appreciation for the diverse characteristics of the generation(s) that comprise the classroom. This is one area of exploration and subsequent professional development that educators might not realize is important. Centers for Teaching and Learning are excellent resources and have a goal to further develop and engage educators at their institution. While the physical location of a center for teaching and learning might be on the periphery of campus, the intent of these centers is holistic and provides centralized support for educators (Sorcinelli 2002).

Students benefit when their teachers are effective educators. As described in Chapter 5, the most highly valued qualities of health profession educators include being approachable, personable, effective communicators, encouraging, caring, enthusiastic, knowledgeable, understanding, and having realistic expectations for classroom learning (Groccia et al. 2018). While being knowledgeable about the subject matter is important, students desire educators with whom they can relate. Centers for teaching and learning offer opportunities for educators to learn techniques that increase their ability to connect with students in humanistic ways. They also create communities of educators who share ideas and collaborate. By connecting those with similar interests, communities are created. These communities, whose members might not naturally interact, enhance the development of one another by idea sharing.

Role of Scholarship of Teaching and Learning for Supporting Long-Term Curricular Changes

The role of higher education is to provide learners with the knowledge, skills, and abilities needed to successfully navigate the field of study in which they have chosen and to foster and promote the role of lifelong learning to further support their careers as they progress through life. As we strive to create lifelong learners in our students, we must accept that as educators we are also tasked with this same charge, to continue learning, adapting, and innovating our own teaching practices. To achieve this goal, we must acknowledge the nuances between being a scholarly teacher and creating the scholarship of teaching and learning (SoTL). Potter and Kustra (2011) denote the connections between the two areas, as well as what distinguishes them from one another. They define scholarly teaching as staying current within the SoTL literature, applying best practices to the teaching and learning environment, the incorporation of peer mentoring, feedback, and critical reflection, with a primary goal of effective teaching to maximize student learning. SoTL, on the other hand, is defined as a systematic approach to studying teaching and learning with the intent to share findings publicly. The ultimate goal of SoTL is to create a better and/or more accurate understanding of factors that maximize learning. Scholarly teachers are the "consumers" of the work created by SoTL scholars, who are "producers" (Mauer 2022). While the end goal is basically the same for scholarly teaching and SoTL, Potter and Kustra posit that scholarly teaching has a more direct influence on learning than does SoTL, though the exact nature of the relationship between the two is more nuanced and continues to be an area for debate (2011).

As educators, sharing best practices within the teaching and learning environment is crucial to support and enhance the academy (Boyer 1990). SoTL and scholarly teaching continue to be important aspects of higher education as it allows faculty to explore alternative strategies for developing, implementing, and evaluating new and innovative approaches within their courses and clinical experiences. SoTL and scholarly teaching also push faculty to critically evaluate if their strategies are effective in accomplishing the goals of the experience but can also encourage faculty to step outside of their comfort zones to try something new, which can lead to positive learning outcomes. Faculty should feel empowered to push not only their students to try something new but themselves as well. The incorporation of innovative teaching strategies can result in happier students and more engaged faculty.

Identifying as a SoTL researcher can be challenging when done in isolation, and the development of SoTL communities both within and outside of the parent institution should support this continuous development. These communities can be formal or informal and can provide the infrastructure needed for long-term and short-term initiatives. For example, the authors of this text have a long-standing community that began when all four scholars were located at one institution. However, these relationships have continued even as members have transitioned to other institutions across the United States. The foundational elements of the community have remained the same, with each member contributing to scholarly projects due to their own unique expertise and work experience.

Integration of Mentoring and Alignment with Positive Outcomes

Strong mentoring relationships and positive role models are essential within the experiential learning environment. As a relational process, mentoring relationships require that both parties be invested in the relationship and to host and maintain open and honest dialogue. The very nature of healthcare requires that teams work effectively, and a key aspect of these teams demands that each member serve as both a mentor and a mentee. To ensure that learners are prepared for these relationships once they transition into practice, they must first experience the mentoring relationship during their academic program.

As educators, it is expected that we train students to emulate the characteristics and behaviors they hope to adopt upon entry into the workforce (Mylrea, Gupta, and Glass 2015). Mentors need to establish lasting connections with their mentees, showcasing the value of a lasting relationship and the benefits of serving as a mentor to others. Furthermore, educators need to ensure that mentees understand that each mentoring dynamic will be different and based on the needs of the two individuals within the relationship. A well-established mentoring relationship will ensure that learners are prepared for the profession and will feel a sense of belonging within their academic program. These positive dynamics have historically resulted in improved outcomes within the program and have eased the transition into practice (Weinberg 2019).

NEXT UP: GENERATION ALPHA

Behind Generation Z comes those born between 2010 and 2025, already labeled as Generation Alpha and projected to number nearly two billion globally (Annie E. Casey Foundation 2020). Children of Millennials and younger siblings of Generation Z, this generation is projected to go to college in greater proportions, potentially boosting a languishing enrollment horizon. Ubiquitous use of technology from birth will result in greater digital literacy and adaptability but also shorter attention spans and delayed social development, important considerations for educators at all levels. They are proposed to be more visual than generations before them and more socially connected through social media outlets. Understanding and accounting for differences in learning style with each new subsequent generation are of paramount importance for educators in all fields, and particularly for those in the health professions.

Conclusion

With the influx of Generation Z learners into higher education, as well as the continued prominence of Millennials in this setting, considerations must be made for creating and maintaining positive learning environments that meet the individual and collective needs of these groups. Educators must remain cognizant of the education landscape to adapt when needed to evolving technology, group dynamics, preferred mode of delivery, innovative pedagogies, and industry standards. Particular attention should also be given to campus resources that meet the needs of students to include increased access, adaptive healthcare delivery modes, and diverse counseling services. This book details these considerations and offers resources for faculty teaching in the health professions who will experience or are already experiencing the shifts that will occur as multigenerational learners matriculate into institutions of higher education.

References

Abu-Rish, Erin, Sara Kim, Lapio Choe, Lara Varpio, Elisabeth Malik, Andrew A White, Karen Craddick, Katherine Blondon, Lynne Robins, Pamela Nagasawa, Allison Thigpen, Lee-Ling Chen, Joanne Rich, and Brenda Zierler. 2012. "Current Trends in Interprofessional Education of Health Sciences Students: A Literature Review." *Journal of Interprofessional Care*, *26*(6): 444–451. https://doi.org/10.3109/13561820.2012.715604.

ACPA: College Student Educators International. 2020. "Statement of Ethical Principles and Standards." *ACPA*. https://myacpa.org/wp-content/uploads/2020/12/Ethical_Principles_Standards.pdf.

Active Minds. 2020. "Creating a Culture of Caring Faculty Resource." https://www.activeminds.org/wp-content/uploads/2020/04/Faculty-Resource_Creating-a-Culture-of-Caring.pdf.

Ahmad, Farida Bhuiya, and Jodi A. Cisewski. 2022. "Quarterly Provisional Estimates for Selected Indicators of Mortality, 2019-Quarter 3, 2021." National Center for Health Statistics. National Vital Statistics System, Vital Statistics Rapid Release Program.

Akin, D., and Lisa M Huang. 2019. "Perceptions of College Students with Disabilities." *Journal of Postsecondary Education and Disability*, *32*(1): 21–33.

Alamuddin, Rayane, Daniel Rossman, and Martin Kurzweil. 2018. "Monitoring Advising Analytics to Promote Success (MAAPS): Evaluation Findings from the First Year of Implementation." Ithaka S+R. https://doi.org/10.18665/sr.307005.

American Association of Colleges of Nursing. 2021. "Competency-Based Education (CBE)." https://www.aacnnursing.org/Portals/42/Downloads/Essentials/CBE-Draft.pdf.

American Association of Colleges of Nursing. 2023. 2022–2023 "Enrollment and Graduations in Baccalaureate and Graduate Programs in Nursing." https://www.aacnnursing.org/store/product-info/productcd/idsr_23enrollbacc.

American Association of Colleges of Pharmacy. 2022. "2021–2022 American Association of Colleges of Pharmacy Competency-Based Education Joint Task Force White Paper." https://connect.aacp.org/viewdocument/competency-based-education-task-for.

American Association of Colleges of Pharmacy. n.d. "Graduating Student." https://www.aacp.org/categories/graduating-student.

American Association of Veterinary Medical Colleges. 2023. "Annual Data Reports." https://www.aavmc.org/about-aavmc/public-data/.

American Council on Education. 1937. *The Student Personnel Point of View.* https://www.naspa.org/files/dmfile/Student_Personnel_Point_of_View_1937.pdf.

American Council on Education. 1949. *The Student Personnel Point of View.* https://www.naspa.org/files/dmfile/Student_Personnel_Point_of_View_1949.pdf.

American Dental Association. 2023. "Why Be a Dentist?" https://www.adea.org/godental/dentistry_101/why_be_a_dentist_.aspx.

American Hospital Association. 2020. "The Value Initiative Issue Brief: Team-Based Care Creates Value." https://www.aha.org/system/files/media/file/2020/09/value-initiative-issue-brief-team-based-care-creates-value.pdf.

The Annie E. Casey Foundation. 2020. "What Is Generation Alpha?" November 4, 2020. https://www.aecf.org/blog/what-is-generation-alpha.

American Pharmacists Association Academy of Students of Pharmacy – American Association of Colleges of Pharmacy Council of Deans Task Force on Professionalism. 2000. "White Paper on Pharmacy Student Professionalism." *Journal of the American Pharmacists Association*, *40*(1): 96–102. https://doi.org/10.1016/S1086-5802(16)31043-9.

American Veterinary Medical Association. 2022. One Health – What Is One Health? https://www.avma.org/resources-tools/one-health.

Aragon, Sofia A., Gerianne M. Babbo, Sarah J. Bear, and Mindy L. Schaffner. 2020. "Nurses at the Table: Action Now! For Nursing Education." *Online Journal of Issues in Nursing*, *25*(1). https://doi.org/10.3912/OJIN.Vol25No01Man04.

Archibald, Robert B., and David H. Feldman. 2018. "Drivers of the Rising Price of a College Education." Midwestern Higher Education Compact. University of Michigan. https://www.mhec.org/sites/default/files/resources/mhec_affordability_series7_20180730_2.pdf.

Armstrong, Shelley, Alison R. McLaughlin, and Jennifer C. Gadarowski. 2021. "Enhancing Competency-Based Education with Virtual Reality Simulation." In Amy deNoyelles, Alyssa Albrecht, Sue Bauer, and Shelly Wyatt (Eds.), *Teaching Online Pedagogical Repository*. Orlando, FL: University of Central Florida Center for Distributed Learning. https://topr.online.ucf.edu/enhancing-competency-based-education-with-virtual-reality-simulation/.

ASPE Office of the Assistant Secretary for Planning and Evaluation. 2002. "Impact of COVID-19 Pandemic on the Hospital and Outpatient Clinician Workforce: Challenges and Policy Response." Retrieved on August 29, 2023, from https://aspe.hhs.gov/sites/default/files/documents/9cc72124abd9ea25d58a22c7692dccb6/aspe-covid-workforce-report.pdf.

Association of American Medical Colleges. 2017. "Table A-6: Age of Applicants to US Medical Schools at Anticipated Matriculation by Sex and Race/Ethnicity, 2014–2015 through 2017–2018." https://www.aamc.org/system/files/d/1/321468-factstablea6.pdf.

Association of American Medical Colleges. 2021. "Table 1: Applicants, Matriculants, Enrollment, and Graduates of U.S. MD-Granting Medical Schools, 2012–2013 through 2021–2022." https://www.aamc.org/media/37816/download?attachment.

Association of American Medical Colleges. 2023. "Group on Student Affairs (GSA)." https://www.aamc.org/career-development/affinity-groups/gsa.

Babiker, Amir, Maha El Husseini, Abdurrahman Al Nemri, Abdurrahman Al Frayh, Nasir Al Juryyan, Mohamed O Faki, Asaad Assiri, Muslim Al Saadi, Farheen Shaikh, and Fahad Al Zamil. 2014. "Health Care Professional Development: Working as a Team to Improve Patient Care." *Sudanese Journal of Paediatrics*, *14*(2): 9–16.

Bailey, Muriel. 2022. BCS "Using Innovative Learning Labs to Break Down Barriers to Inclusion." ABC 33/40 News. https://abc3340.com/news/local/bcs-using-innovative-learning-labs-to-breakdown-barriers-to-digital-inclusion.

Banakou, Domna, Parasuram D. Hanumanthu, and Mel Slater. 2016. "Virtual Embodiment of White People in a Black Virtual Body Leads to a Sustained Reduction in Their Implicit Racial Bias." *Frontiers in Human Neuroscience* 10: 601. https://doi.org/10.3389/fnhum.2016.00601.

Barr, Hugh, Jenny Ford, Richard Gray, Marion Helme, Maggie Hutchings, Helena Low, Alison Machin, and Scott Reeves. 2017. CAIPE 2017 Interprofessional Education Guidelines 2, Center for the Advancement of Interprofessional Education. https://www.caipe.org/resources/publications/caipe-publications/caipe-2017-interprofessional-education-guidelines-barr-h-ford-j-gray-r-helme-m-hutchings-m-low-h-machin-reeves-s.

Beetham, Tamara, David Fiellin, and Susan Busch. 2022. "Physician Response to COVID-19–Driven Telehealth Flexibility for Opioid Use Disorder." *The American Journal of Managed Care*, *28*(9): 456–463. https://doi.org/10.37765/ajmc.2022.89221.

Bergson-Shilcock, Amanda. 2020. "The New Landscape of Digital Literacy." National Skills Coalition. https://www.nationalskillscoalition.org/resource/publications/the-new-landscape-of-digital-literacy/.

Bernhard, Blythe. 2020. "As Non-traditional Students Become the New Norm, Colleges Must Support Generational Diversity." https://www.insightintodiversity.com/as-nontraditional-students-become-the-new-norm-colleges-must-support-generational-diversity/.

Bhatnagar, Vikrant, Sebastian Diaz, and Philip A. Bucur. 2020. "The Need for More Mentorship in Medical School." *Cureus*, *12*(5). https://doi.org/10.7759/cureus.7984.

Bhushan, Alok, Kimberly B. Garza, Omathanu Perumal, Sudip K. Das, David J. Feola, Dorothy Farrell, and Angela Birnbaum. 2022. "Lessons Learned from the COVID-19 Pandemic and Implications for Pharmaceutical Graduate Education and Research." In C. Ford and K. Garza (Eds.), *Handbook of Research on Updating and Innovating Health Professions Education: Post-Pandemic Perspectives* (pp. 324–345). IGI Global. http://doi.org/10.4018/978-1-7998-7623-6.ch014.

Bierer, S. Beth, Elaine F. Dannefer, Christine Taylor, Phillip Hall, and Alan L. Hull. 2008. "Methods to Assess Students' Acquisition, Application and Integration of

Basic Science Knowledge in an Innovative Competency-Based Curriculum." *Medical Teacher*, *30*(7): e171–e177. https://doi.org/10.1080/01421590802139740.

Biggs, John, and Catherine Tang. 2011. *Teaching for Quality Learning at University*. Maidenhead, UK: McGraw-Hill Education.

Birden, Hudson, Nel Glass, Ian Wilson, Michelle Harrison, Tim Usherwood, and Duncan Nass. 2014. "Defining Professionalism in Medical Education: A Systematic Review." *Medical Teacher*, *36*(1): 47–61. https://doi.org/10.3109/0142159X.2014.850154.

Birkenshaw, Julian. n.d. "Beyond the information Age." *Wired Magazine*. Accessed August 31, 2023. https://www.wired.com/insights/2014/06/beyond-information-age/.

Bittner, Aubrey. 2019. "Mentoring Millennials for Nursing Leadership." *Nursing*, *49*(10): 53–56. https://doi.org/10.1097/01.NURSE.0000580656.81188.ee.

Borough of Manhattan Community College. n.d. "Accelerated Study in Associate Programs (ASAP)." https://www.bmcc.cuny.edu/academics/success-programs/asap/.

Bowen, Jose Antonio. 2012. *Teaching Naked*. San Francisco, CA: Jossey Bass.

Boyer, Ernest L. 1990. *Scholarship Reconsidered: Priorities of the Professoriate*. Princeton, NJ: Carnegie Foundation for the Advancement of Teaching.

Boyle, Cynthia J., Robert S. Beardsley, Jill A. Morgan, and Magaly Rodriguez de Bittner. 2007. "Professionalism: A Determining Factor in Experiential Learning." *American Journal of Pharmacy Education*, *71*(2): Article 31. https://doi.org/10.5688/aj710231.

Bradberry, Leigh A., and Jennifer De Maio. 2019. "Learning by Doing: The Long-Term Impact of Experiential Learning Programs on Student Success." *Journal of Political Science Education*, *15*(1): 94–111. https://doi.org/10.1080/15512169.2018.1485571.

Bral, Conna, and Jennifer Cunningham. 2016. "Foundations of Quality in Competency-Based Programs: Competencies and Assessments." *The Journal of Competency-Based Education*, *1*(3): 118–121. https://doi.org/10.1002/cbe2.1027.

Brant, Katarina, and Stephanie L. Castro. 2019. "You Can't Ignore Millennials: Needed Changes and a New Way Forward in Entitlement Research." *Human Resource Management Journal*, *29*(4): 527–538. https://doi.org/10.1111/1748-8583.12262.

Branzetti, Jeremy, Michael A. Gisondi, Laura R. Hopson, and Linda Regan. 2019. "Aiming beyond Competent: The Application of the Taxonomy of Significant Learning to Medical Education." *Teaching and Learning in Medicine*, *31*(4): 466–478. https://doi.org/10.1080/10401334.2018.1561368.

Bric, Justin D., Derek C. Lumbard, Matthew J. Frelich, and Jon C. Gould. 2016. "Current State of Virtual Reality Simulation in Robotic Surgery Training: A Review." *Surgical Endoscopy*, *30*(6): 2169–2178. https://doi.org/10.1007/s00464-015-4517-y.

Bridges, Diane R., Richard A. Davidson, Peggy Soule Odegard, Ivan V. Maki, and John Tomkowiak. 2011. "Interprofessional Collaboration: Three Best Practice Models of Interprofessional Education." *Medical Education Online*, *16*(1): 6035. https://doi.org/10.3402/meo.v16i0.6035.

Broadsky, Sascha. September 26, 2022. "How AI writing Tools Are Helping Students Fake Their Own Homework." *Lifewire*. https://www.lifewire.com/how-ai-writing-tools-are-helping-students-fake-their-homework-6743857.

Brown, Sarah. 2022. "How Generations X, Y, and Z May Change the Academic Workplace." The Chronicle of Higher Education. June 14, 2022. https://www.chronicle.com/article/how-generations-x-y-and-z-may-change-the-academic-workplace/.

Burke, Lilah. 2021. "A 'Fauci Effect'?" *Inside Higher Ed*. https://www.insidehighered.com/admissions/article/2021/01/11/health-professions-schools-see-surge-applications.

Busteed, Brandon. 2020. "8 Innovative Ideas for Higher Education Right Now." *Forbes*. https://www.forbes.com/sites/brandonbusteed/2020/07/23/8-innovative-ideas-for-higher-education-right-now/?sh=3c107fa96496.

Caplan, Zoe. May 25, 2023. "U.S. Older Population Grew from 2010 to 2020 at Fastest Rate since 1880 to 1890." Census.gov. https://www.census.gov/library/stories/2023/05/2020-census-united-states-older-population-grew.html#:~:text=In%202020%2C%20the%20bulge%20is,is%20projected%20to%20start%20slowing.

Carlson, Keith. 2023. "Is Nursing School Worth It?" *Nurse Journal*. https://nursejournal.org/resources/is-a-nursing-degree-worth-it/.

Chamberlain, Samuel. 2023. "Supreme Court Outlaws Affirmative Action in College Admissions in Landmark Decision." *New York Post*. https://nypost.com/2023/06/29/supreme-court-outlaws-affirmative-action-in-college-admissions/.

Chen, Po-Ju, and Youngsoo Choi. 2008. "Generational Difference in Work Values: A Study of Hospitality Management." *International Journal of Contemporary Hospital Management*, *20*(6): 595–615. https://doi.org/10.1108/09596110810892182.

Chicca, Jennifer, and Teresa Shellenbarger. 2018. "Connecting with Generation Z: Approaches in Nursing Education." *Teaching and Learning in Nursing*, *13*(3): 180–184. https://doi.org/10.1016/j.teln.2018.03.008.

Chickering, Arthur W., and Linda Reisser. 1993. "The Seven Vectors." In *Education and Identity*, second edition, 34–52. San Francisco: Jossey-Bass.

Chidiac, Joseph E, Ahmed Mohamed, Madhumitha Krishnamoorthy, Karim Mahmoud, Geethapriya Rajasekaranrathnakumar, Mohan Palla, and Diane L Levine. 2018. "US Medical Schools' Awareness of Their Students Who Smoke, Cessation Programs Available, and the Potential Impact on Residency Match." *Nicotine & Tobacco Research*, *20*(6): 785. https://doi.org/10.1093/ntr/ntx174.

Chiu, Chia-Ju. 2014. "Development and Validation of Performance Assessment Tools for Interprofessional Communication and Teamwork (PACT)." PhD diss., University of Washington.

Chory, Rebecca M., and Evan H. Offstein. 2017. "'Your Professor Will Know You as a Person': Evaluating and Rethinking the Relational Boundaries between Faculty and Students." *Journal of Management Education*, *41*(1): 9–38. https://doi.org/10.1177/1052562916647986.

Cleary, Michelle Navarre, and Catherine Breathnach. 2017. "Competency-Based Education as a Force for Equity." *Journal of Competency-Based Education* 2: e01040. https://doi.org/10.1002/cbe2.1040.

Comeveo. 2018. "Higher Education Recruitment Strategies for Gen Z." August 22, 2018. https://comevo.com/higher-education-recruitment-strategies-gen-z/.

Coomes, Michael D., and Robert DeBard. 2004. "A Generational Approach to Understanding Students." *New Directions for Teaching and Learning*, *106*(Summer): 5–16. https://doi.org/10.1002/ss.121.

Cooper, Michelle. 2022. "What Impact Does the Nursing Shortages Have on the Financial Health of the Kentucky Healthcare System?" MPA/MPP/MPFM Capstone Projects, 353. https://uknowledge.uky.edu/mpampp_etds/353.

Cornine, Amanda. 2020. "Reducing Nursing Student Anxiety in the Clinical Setting: An Integrative Review." *Nursing Education Perspectives*, *41*(4): 229–234. https://doi.org/10.1097/01.NEP.0000000000000633.

Council for the Advancement of Standards. 2006. "CAS Statement of Shared Ethical Principles." In *CAS Professional Standards for Higher Education*, Washington, DC: Author. https://www.cas.edu/files/CASethicsstatement.pdf.

Council on Social Work Education. 2015. "Education and Policy Accreditation Standards." https://www.cswe.org/Accreditation/Standards-and-Policies/2015-EPAS.

Council on Social Work Education. 2022. "Education and Policy Accreditation Standards." https://www.cswe.org/getmedia/94471c42-13b8-493b-9041-b30f48533d64/2022-EPAS.pdf.

Courtenay, Molly, Joelle Sweeney, Paulina Zielinska, Sarah Brown Blake, and Roberto La Ragione. 2015. "One Health: An Opportunity for an Interprofessional Approach to Healthcare." *Journal of Interprofessional Care*, *29*(6): 641–642. https://doi.org/10.3109/13561820.2015.1041584.

Cox, Jesse, and Madison Holloway. 2011. "Workshop on Knowledge Transfer in a Multigenerational Business Environment." *Review of Management Innovation and Creativity*, *4*(10): 23–33.

Cruess, Richard L., Sylvia R. Cruess, Donald Boudreau, Linda Snell, and Yvonne Steinert. 2014. "Reframing Medical Education to Support Professional Identity Formation." *Academic Medicine*, *89*(11): 1446–1451. https://doi.org/10.1097/ACM.0000000000000047.

Cruess, Richard L., Sylvia R. Cruess. J. Donald Boudreau, Linda Snell, Yvonne Steinert. 2015. "A Schematic Representation of the Professional Identity Formation and Socialization of Medical Students and Residents: A Guide for Medical Educators." *Academic Medicine*, *90*(6): 718–725. https://doi.org/10.1097/ACM.0000000000000700.

Cruess, Richard L., Sylvia R. Cruess, and Yvonne Steinert. 2016. "Amending Miller's Pyramid to Include Professional Identity Formation." *Academic Medicine*, *91*(2): 180–185. https://doi.org/10.1097/ACM.0000000000000913.

Cruess, Sylvia R., Richard L. Cruess, and Yvonne Steinert. 2019. "Supporting the Development of a Professional Identity: General Principles." *Medical Teacher*, *41*(6): 641–649. https://doi.org/10.1097/ACM.0000000000000700.

Dall'Alba, Gloria. 2009. "Learning Professional Ways of Being: Ambiguities of Becoming." *Educational Philosophy and Theory*, *41*(1): 34–45. https://doi.org/10.1111/j.1469-5812.2008.00475.x.

Daugherty, Terry, and Ernest Hoffman. 2014. "eWOM and the Importance of Capturing Consumer Attention within Social Media." *Journal of Marketing Communications*, *20*(1–2): 82–102. https://doi.org/10.1080/13527266.2013.797764.

Dawson, Rachel Fulcher, Melissa S. Kearney, and James X. Sullivan. 2021a. "Comprehensive Approaches to Increasing Student Completion in Higher Education: A Survey of the Landscape." In *National Bureau of Economic Research*. NBER Working Paper Series, 28046.

Dawson, Rachel Fulcher, Melissa S. Kearney, and James X. Sullivan. 2021b. "Why Expanded Student Supports Can Improve Community College Outcomes and Boost Skill Attainment." The Brookings Institution. https://www.brookings.edu/blog/brown-center-chalkboard/2021/04/07/why-expanded-student-supports-can-improve-community-college-outcomes-and-boost-skill-attainment/.

Delgado, Danielle, Noreen Hill, Ana Regalado, and Nicolle Waldman. 2020. "Millennials Leading the Workforce." *Journal of Business Studies Quarterly*, *10*(2): 35–42.

Destoumieux-Garzón, Delphine, Patrick Mavingui, Giles Boetsch, Jérôme Boissier, Frédéric Darriet, Priscilla Duboz, Clémentine Fritsch, Patrick Giraudoux, Frédérique Le Roux, Serge Morand, Christine Paillard, Dominique Pontier, Cédric Sueur, and Yann Voituron. 2018. "The One Health Concept: 10 Years Old and a Long Road Ahead." *Frontiers in Veterinary Science*, *5*: 14. https://doi.org/10.3389/fvets.2018.00014.

Desy, Janeve R., Darcy A. Reed, and Alexandra P. Wolanskyj. 2017. "Milestones and Millennials: A Perfect Pairing – Competency-Based Medical Education and the Learning Preferences of Generation Y." *Mayo Clinic Proceedings*, *92*(2): 243–250. https://doi.org/10.1016/j.mayocp.2016.10.026.

De Villiers, M. Ruth. 2006. "A Learning Theory Approach in Support of Outcomes-Based e-Learning." CITTE 2006 Conference on Information Technology in Tertiary Education.

Dewsbury, Bryan M. 2017. "Context Determines Strategies for 'Activating' the Inclusive Classroom." *Journal of Microbiology & Biology Education*, *18*(3). https://doi.org/10.1128/jmbe.v18i3.1347.

Dewsbury, Bryan M., and Cynthia J. Brame. 2019. "Inclusive Teaching." *CBE – Life Science Education*, *18*(2): 1–5. https://doi.org/10.1187/cbe.19-01-0021

Dickie, R. 2016. "History of Interprofessional Education. Interprofessional Education and Medical Libraries: Partnering For Success." In *Interprofessional Education and Medical Libraries: Partnering for Success*, edited by Mary Edwards, 1–11. Lanham, MD: Rowman and Littlefiled.

Dickler, Jessica. 2021. "Post-Pandemic, the Office Will Have a Whole New Look." *CNBC Personal Finance*, July 12, 2021. https://www.cnbc.com/2021/07/12/post-pandemic-offices-have-a-new-look-as-employers-adopt-hoteling.html.

Dominguez, Daniel G., David S. Fike, Eric J. MacLaughlin, and Joseph A. Zorek. 2015. A Comparison of the Validity of Two Instruments Assessing Health Professional Student Perceptions of Interprofessional Education and Practice." *Journal of Interprofessional Care*, *29*(2): 144–149. https://doi.org/10.3109/13561820.2014.94.

Douglas, Mark, Tim Howell, Elaine Nelson, Laurel Pilkington, and Irene Salinas. 2015. "Improve the Function of Multigenerational Teams." *Nursing Management*, *46*(1): 11–13. https://doi.org/10.1097/01.NUMA.0000459098.71482.c4.

Dungy, Gwendolyn Jordan. 2018. "Students and Student Affairs: Facing Perennial Challenges in Ever-Changing Contexts." *Change: The Magazine of Higher Learning*, *50*(3–4): 58–62. https://doi.org/10.1080/00091383.2018.1509600.

Duquesne University School of Nursing. 2022. "The Shortage of Healthcare Workers in the U.S." https://onlinenursing.duq.edu/post-master-certificates/shortage-of-healthcare-workers/.

Dyer, Elizabeth, Barbara J. Swartzlander, and Marilyn R. Gugliucci. 2018. "Using Virtual Reality in Medical Education to Teach Empathy." *Journal of the Medical Library Association: JMLA*, *106*(4): 498–500. https://doi.org/10.5195/jmla.2018.518.

Dyrbye, Liselotte N., Matthew R. Thomas, F. Stanford Massie, David V. Power, Anne Eacker, William Harper, Steven Durning, Christine Moutier, Daniel W. Szydlo, Paul J. Novotny, Jeff A. Sloan, and Tait D. Shanafelt. 2008. "Burnout and Suicidal Ideation among US Medical Students." *Annals of Internal Medicine*, *149*(5): 334–341. https://doi.org/10.7326/0003-4819-149-5-200809020-00008.

Dyrbye, Liselotte N., William Harper, Steven J. Durning, Christine Moutier, Matthew R. Thomas, F. Stanford Massie Jr., Anne Eacker, David V. Power, Daniel W. Szydlo, Jeff A. Sloan, and Tait D. Shanafelt. 2011. "Patterns of Distress in US Medical Students." *Medical Teacher*, *33*(10): 834–839. https://doi.org/10.3109/0142159X.2010.531158.

EAB. 2018. "Move Over, Millennials. Gen Z Is Coming to the Workforce." EAB. July 18, 2018. https://eab.com/insights/daily-briefing/workplace/move-over-millennials-gen-z-is-coming-to-the-workforce/.

Eckleberry-Hunt, Jodie, David Lick, and Ronald Hunt. 2018. "Is Medical Education Ready for Generation Z?" *Journal of Graduate Medical Education*, *10*(4): 378–381. https://doi.org/10.4300/JGME-D-18-00466.1.

Educause. n.d. "The Digital versus Brick-and-Mortar Balancing Game." https://www.educause.edu/showcase-series/2022/the-digital-versus-brick-and-mortar-balancing-game.

Eisenberg, Daniel, Ezra Golberstein, and Justin Hunt. 2009. "Mental Health and Academic Success in College." *The B.E. Journal of Economic Analysis & Policy*, *9*(1): Article 40. https://doi.org/10.2202/1935-1682.2191.

Evans, Retta R., and Laura Forbes. 2012. "Mentoring the 'Net Generation': Faculty Perspectives in Health Education." *College Student Journal*, *46*(2): 397–405.

Fedele, Robert. 2020. "Behind Angry Stan, the Virtual Reality Simulator Training Nursing Students to Deal with Conflict." *Australian Nursing and Midwifery Journal*, March 27, 2020. https://anmj.org.au/behind-angry-stan-the-virtual-reality-simulator-training-nursing-students-to-deal-with-conflict/.

Federal Reserve Economic Database. 2023. "S&P/Case-Shiller US National Home Price Index. "https://fred.stlouisfed.org/series/CSUSHPISA.

Feldmann, John. 2022. "The Double Standard of Post-Pandemic Employee Benefits." *Forbes Human Resources Council*, June 10, 2022. https://www.forbes.com/sites/

forbeshumanresourcescouncil/2022/06/10/the-double-standard-of-post-pandemic-employee-benefits/?sh=5ac307f73b7b.

Felten, Peter, and Leo M. Lambert. 2020. *Relationship-Rich Education: How Human Connections Drive Success in College*. Baltimore, MD: Johns Hopkins University Press.

Fertleman, Caroline, Phoebe Aubugeau-Williams, Carmel Sher, Ai-Nee Lim, Sophie Lumley, Sylvi Delacroix and Xueni Pan. 2018. "A Discussion of Virtual Reality as a New Tool for Training Healthcare Professionals." *Frontiers in Public Health*, *6*: 44. https://doi.org/10.3389/fpubh.2018.00044.

Fewster-Thuente, Lori and Tamzin J. Batteson. 2018. "Kolb's Experiential Learning Theory as a Theoretical Underpinning for Interprofessional Education." *Journal of Allied Health Professions*, *47*(1): 3–8.

Field, Kelly. 2021a. "The Mental Health Challenge." In *Recruiting and Retaining Students in a Challenging Market*, edited by Kelly Field, Eric Kelderman, Katherine Mangan, and Brian O'Leary, 56–67. The Chronicle of Higher Education. https://store.chronicle.com/products/recruiting-and-retaining-students-in-a-challenging-market.

Field, Kelly. 2021b. "The Missing Men." *Chronicle of Higher Education*. https://www.chronicle.com/article/the-missing-men.

Field, Kelly, Eric Kelderman, Katherine Mangan, and Brian O'Leary. 2021. *Recruiting and Retaining Students in a Challenging Market*. The Chronicle of Higher Education. https://store.chronicle.com/products/recruiting-and-retaining-students-in-a-challenging-market.

Fink, L. Dee. 2013. *Creating Significant Learning Experiences: An Integrated Approach to Designing College Courses*. San Francisco, CA: Jossey-Bass.

Finley, Ashley. 2021. "How College Contributes to Workforce Success: Employer Views on What Matters Most." Hanover Research. https://files.eric.ed.gov/fulltext/ED616977.pdf.

Finn, Amber N., Paul Schrodt, Paul L. Witt, Nikki Elledge, Kodiane A. Jernberg, and Lara M. Larson. 2009. "A Meta-Analytical Review of Teacher Credibility and Its Associations with Teacher Behaviors and Student Outcomes." *Communication Education*, *58*(4): 516–537. https://doi.org/10.1080/03634520903131154.

Fischer, Karin. 2021. "More International Grad Students Wanted to Come to the U.S., but Couldn't." *The Chronicle of Higher Education*, February 18, 2021. https://www.chronicle.com/article/more-international-grad-students-wanted-to-come-to-the-u-s-but-couldnt.

Fitzgerald, Anita. 2020. "Professional Identity: A Concept Analysis." In *Nursing Forum*, *55*(3): 447–472.

Flaherty, Ellen, and Bartels, Stephen J. 2019. "Addressing the Community-Based Geriatric Healthcare Workforce Shortage by Leveraging the Potential of Interprofessional Teams." *Journal of the American Geriatrics Society*, *67*(52): s400-s408. https://doi.org/10.1111/jgs.15924.

Flanagan, E. 2022. "Effective Soft Skills (or Should We Say 'Power Skills') Explained." *Unboxed Training and Technology*, April 4, 2022. https://www.unboxedtechnology.com/blog/what-are-power-skills/.

Ford, Channing R., and Erika L. Kleppinger. 2020. "Designing, Implementing, and Evaluating Performance-Based Assessments within a Competency-Driven Curriculum." In *Cases on Instructional Design and Performance Outcomes in Medical Education*, edited by Jill Stefaniak, 183–209. Hershey, PA: IGI Global. https://doi.org/10.4018/978-1-7998-5092-2.ch009.

Ford, Channing R., and Lindsey Moseley. 2020. "Challenges to Health Professions Education and Strategies for Moving Forward." In *Innovative Teaching and Learning in the Health Professions*," edited by Channing R. Ford and James E. Groccia. *New Directions for Teaching and Learning*, *162*: 199–207. https://doi.org/10.1002/tl.20404.

Ford, Jenny, and Richard Gray. 2021. *Interprofessional Education Handbook: Center for the Advancement of Interprofessional Education.* Centre for the Advancement of Interprofessional Education. https://www.caipe.org/resources/publications/caipe-publications/caipe-2021-a-new-caipe-interprofessional-education-handbook-2021-ipe-incorporating-values-based-practice-ford-j-gray-r.

Frahm, Josh. 2019. "Engaging Generation Z." *NACE Blog*, November 12, 2019. https://community.naceweb.org/blogs/josh-frahm1/2019/11/12/engaging-generation-z.

Frank, Jason R., Linda S. Snell, Olle Ten Cate, Eric S. Holmboe, Carol Carraccio, Susan R. Swing, Peter Harris, et al. 2010. "Competency-Based Medical Education: Theory to Practice." *Medical* Teacher, *32*(8): 638–645. https://doi.org/10.3109/0142159X.2010.501190.

Frank, Jason R, Sarah Taber, Marta van Zanten, Fedde Scheele, and Danielle Blouin. 2020. "The Role of Accreditation in 21st Century Health Professions Education: Report of an International Consensus Group." *BMC Medical Education*, *20* (Suppl 1): 305. https://doi.org/10.1186/s12909-020-02121-5.

Fry, Richard. 2018. "Millennials Are the Largest Generation in the U.S. Labor Force." Pew Research Center, April 11, 2018. https://www.pewresearch.org/fact-tank/2018/04/11/millennials-largest-generation-us-labor-force/.

Garza, Kimberly B., Brandy R. Davis, Alexicia Richardson, Cheryl Seals, Chad G. Rose, Gary Hawkins, and Adelia Grabowsky. 2023. "Walking in Their Shoes: Using Virtual Reality to Promote Empathy for Patients among Student Pharmacists." Poster presentation at the American Association of Colleges of Pharmacy Annual Meeting, July 2023, Aurora, CO.

Gaspar, Connor, and Cindy Waxer. n.d. "Generation Z Behavior: Let's Make a Difference but Also Watch What Celebrities Buy." *SAP Insights.* https://insights.sap.com/generation-z-behavior-explained/.

Gerhardt, Megan, Josephine Nachemson-Ekwall, and Brandon Fogel. 2021. *Gentelligence: The Revolutionary Approach to Leading an Intergenerational Workforce*. Lanham, MD: Rowman & Littlefield.

Gervais, Jennifer. 2016. "The Operational Definition of Competency-based Education." *The Journal of Competency-Based Education*, *1*(2): 98–106. https://doi.org/10.1002/cbe2.1011.

Giancola, Frank. 2006. "The Generation Gap: More Myth than Reality." *Human Resource Planning*, *29*(4): 32–37.

Gilbert, John H. V., Jean Yan, and Steven J. Hoffman. 2010. "A WHO report: Framework for Action on Interprofessional Education and Collaborative Practice." *Journal of Allied Health*, *39*(Suppl 1): 196–197.

Gillespie, Gordon Lee, Sharon Farra, Saundra L. Rega, and Susan V. Brammer. 2021. "Impact of Immersive Virtual Reality Simulations for Changing Knowledge, Attitudes, and Behaviors." *Nurse Education Today*, *105*(2021): 105025. https://doi.org/10.1016/j.nedt.2021.105025.

Goh, Hongli Sam, Hui Zhang, Chen Na Lee, Xi Vivien Wu, and Wenru Wang. 2019. "Value of Nursing Objective Structured Clinical Examinations: A Scoping Review." *Nursing Educator*, *44*(5): E1–E6. https://doi.org/10.1097/NNE/0000000000000620.

Gopalan, Maithreyi, Ashley Linden-Carmichael, and Stephanie Lanza. 2022. "College Students' Sense of Belonging and Mental Health amidst the COVID-19 Pandemic." *Journal of Adolescent Health*, *70*(2): 228–33. https://doi.org/10.1016/j.jadohealth.2021.10.010.

Grace, Sandra, Ev Innes, Narelle Patton, and Lynette Stockhausen. 2017. "Ethical Experiential Learning in Medical, Nursing and Allied Health Education: A Narrative Review." *Nurse Education Today*, *51*: 23–33. https://doi.org/10.1016/j.nedt.2016.12.024.

Gramlich, John. 2017. "Hispanic Dropout Rate Hits New Low, College Enrollment at New High." Pew Research Center, September 29, 2017. https://www.pewresearch.org/fact-tank/2017/09/29/hispanic-dropout-rate-hits-new-low-college-enrollment-at-new-high/.

Grawe, Nathan D. 2018. Demographics and the Demand for Higher Education. Baltimore: Johns Hopkins University Press.

Greico, Christina. 2020. "SoTL Showcase: Accessible Assignments through Document Design (abstract)." *Teaching Towards the Future*, *12*(2020). https://doi.org/10.13021/itlcp.2020.2770.

Grice, Gloria R., Angela R. Thomason, Lisa M. Meny, Nicole R. Pinelli, Jay L. Martello, and Joseph A. Zorek. 2018. "Intentional Interprofessional Experiential Education." *American Journal of Pharmaceutical Education*, *82*(3): 6502. https://doi.org/10.5688/ajpe6502.

Groccia, James E., Emad A Ismail, Mary McConner, Channing R. Ford, and Kelley Noll. 2018. "Perceptions of Excellent Teachers: International, HBCU, and Health Professions Perspectives." In *Habits and Practices of Master Teachers: International Perspectives on Excellent Teaching*, edited by William Buskist and Jared W. Keeley. *New Directions for Teaching and Learning* 2018 (156): 85–94. https://doi.org/10.1002/tl.20320.

Hallowell, Edward M., and John J. Ratey. 2011. *Driven to Distraction (revised): Recognizing and Coping with Attention Deficit Disorder*. New York: Anchor.

Hamilton Brady E., Joyce A. Martin, and Michelle J. K. Osterman. 2021. "Births: Provisional Data for 2020." *Vital Statistics Rapid Release*, *12*: 1–11. https://doi.org/10.15620/cdc:104993.

Hamilton, Erica R., Joshua M. Rosenberg, and Mete Akcaoglu. 2016. "The Substitution Augmentation Modification Redefinition (SAMR) Model: A Critical Review and Suggestions for its Use." *TechTrends*, *60*: 433–441. https://doi.org/10.1007/s11528-016-0091-y.

Hammer, Dana P., Bruce A. Berger, R. S. Beardsley, and Michelle R. Easton. 2003. "Student Professionalism." *American Journal of Pharmaceutical Education*, *67*(3): Article 96.

Hammick, Marilyn, Della Freeth, Ivan Koppel, Scott Reeves, and Hugh Barr. 2007. "A Best Evidence Systematic Review of Interprofessional Education: BEME Guide no. 9." *Medical Teacher*, *29*(8): 735–751. https://doi.org/10.1080/01421590701682576.

Hampton, Debbie C., and Yolanda Keys. 2016. "Generation Z Students: Will They Change Our Nursing Classrooms?" *Journal of Nursing Education and Practice*, *7*(4): 111–115. https://doi.org/10.5430/jnep.v7n4p111.

Han, Sang G., Young C. Kim, Tae Y. Kong, and Junho Cho. 2021. "Virtual Reality-Based Neurological Examination Teaching Tool (VRNET) versus Standardized Patient in Teaching Neurological Examinations for the Medical Students: A Randomized, Single-blind Study." *BMC Medical Education*, *21*(1): 493. https://doi.org/10.1186/s12909-021-02920-4.

Hanson, Melanie. 2022. "College Enrollment and Student Demographic Statistics." Education Data Initiative. Last modified July 26, 2022. https://educationdata.org/college-enrollment-statistics.

Harden, Ronald M. 1988. "What Is an OSCE?" *Medical Teacher*, *10*(1): 19–22. https://doi.org/10.3109/01421598809019321.

Harden, Ronald M., and F. A. Gleeson. 1979. "ASME Medical Education Booklet No. 8, Assessment of Medical Competence Using an Objective Structured Clinical Examination (OSCE)." *Medical Education*, *13*(1): 41–54. https://doi.org/10.1111/j.1365-2923.1979.tb00918.x.

Harrington, Cuan M., Dara O. Kavanagh, John F. Quinlan, Donncha Ryan, Patrick Dicker, Dara O'Keeffe, Oscar Traynor, and Sean Tierney. 2018. "Development and Evaluation of a Trauma Decision-Making Simulator in Oculus Virtual Reality." *American Journal of Surgery*, *215*(1): 42–47. https://doi.org/10.1016/j.amjsurg.2017.02.011.

Harris, P., Snell, L., Talbot, M., Harden, R. M. 2010. "Competency-Based Medical Education: Implications for Undergraduate Programs." *Medical Teacher*, *32*(8): 646–650. https://doi.org/10.3109/0142159X.2010.500703.

Harvey, Bryan C. 2021. "Teetering on the Demographic Cliff, Part 1: Prepare Now for the Challenging Times Ahead." *Planning for Higher Education*, *49*(4): 1–13.

Health Professions Accreditors Collaborative. 2019. Guidance on Developing Quality Interprofessional Education for the Health Professions. https://healthprofessionsaccreditors.org//wp-content/uploads/2019/02/HPACGuidance02-01-19.pdf.

HelloCampus. 2022. "How Generation Z Views Higher Education." https://hellocampus.com/post/how-generation-z-views-higher-education.

Herrera, Fernanda, Jeremy Bailenson, Erika Weisz, Elise Ogle, and Jamil Zaki. 2018. "Building Long-Term Empathy: A Large-Scale Comparison of Traditional and

Virtual Reality Perspective-Taking." *PLoS ONE, 13*(10): e0204494. https://doi.org/10.1371/journal.pone.0204494.

Hew, Khe Foo, and Chung Kwan Lo. 2018. "Flipped Classroom Improves Student Learning in Health Professions Education: A Meta-Analysis." *BMC Medical Education, 18*(38): 1–12. https://doi.org/10.1186/s12909-018-1144-z.

Hirsch, Ariel E., Ankit Agarwal, Alexander E. Rand, Nicholas J. DeNunzio, Krishnan R. Patel, Minh Tam Truong, Gregory A. Russo, and Lisa A. Kachnic. 2014. "Medical Student Mentorship in Radiation Oncology at a Single Academic Institution: A 10-Year Analysis." *Practical Radiation Oncology*, *5*(3): E163-E168. https://doi.org/10.1016/j.prro.2014.08.005.

Hodges, Ashley L., Annette Jakubisin Konicki, Michele H. Talley, Curry J. Bordelon, Aimee C. Holland, and F. Shawn Galin. 2019. "Competency-Based Education in Transitioning Nurse Practitioner Students from Education to Practice." *Journal of the American Association of Nurse Practitioners, 31*(2019): 675–682. https://doi.org/10.1097/JXX.0000000000000327.

Holden, Mark D., Era Buck, John Luk, Frank Ambriz, Eugene V. Boisaubin, Mark A. Clark, Angela P. Mihalic, John Z. Sadler, Kenneth J. Sapire, Jeffrey P. Spike, Alan Vince, and John L. Dalrymple. 2015. "Professional Identity Formation: Creating a Longitudinal Framework through TIME (Transformation in Medical Education)." *Academic Medicine*, *90*(6): 761–767. https://doi.org/10.1097/ACM.0000000000000719.

Holzer, Harry J. 2015. "Higher Education and Workforce Policy: Creating More Skilled Workers (and Jobs for Them to Fill)." The Brookings Institution, April 6, 2015. https://www.brookings.edu/research/higher-education-and-workforce-policy-creating-more-skilled-workers-and-jobs-for-them-to-fill/.

Howe, Neil, and William Strauss. 2000. *Millennials Rising: The Next Great Generation.* New York: Vintage Books.

Howe, Neil, and William Strauss. 2003. *Millennials Go to College: Strategies for a New Generation on Campus.* Washington, DC: American Association of Collegiate Registrars and Admissions Officers and LifeCourse Associates.

Hugus, Erin, Mary Tkatchov, Brianna K. Becker, Kendra Hunter, and G. Blue Brazelton. 2021. "Lessons for the Future: Learning from Virtual Student Services." In *Virtual Delivery of Student Services – Post Covid*, edited by G. Blue Brazelton, Erin Hugus, Mary Tkatachov, Kendra Hunter, and Brianna K. Becker. *New Directions for Student Services, 2021*(176): 81–85. https://doi.org/10.1002/ss.20408.

Hyder, Maryam A., and Junaid Razzak. 2020. "Telemedicine in the United States: An Introduction for Students and Residents." *Journal of Medical Internet Research, 22*(11): e20839. https://doi.org/10.2196/20839.

Inside Track. n.d. Accessed December 15, 2022. https://www.insidetrack.org/.

Institute of International Education (IIE). 2020. *Open Doors: Report on International Educational Exchange*. Washington, DC: IIE. https://opendoorsdata.org/.

Institute of Medicine. 2004. *In the Nation's Compelling Interest: Ensuring Diversity in the Health-Care Workforce.* Washington, DC: The National Academies Press. https://doi.org/10.17226/10885.

Institute of Medicine Committee on Health Professions, Education Summit. 2003. *Health Professions Education: A Bridge to Quality.* Washington, DC: The National Academies Press. https://nap.nationalacademies.org/catalog/10681/health-professions-education-a-bridge-to-quality.

Institute of Medicine Committee on the Health Professions, Education Interprofessional Education Collaborative (IPEC). 2016. "Core Competencies for Interprofessional Collaborative Practice: Report of an Expert Panel." Washington, DC: Interprofessional Education Collaborative. http://www.asha.org/uploadedFiles/Interprofessional-Collaboration-Core-Competency.pdf.

Institute of Medicine Committee on Quality of Health Care in America. 2001. *Crossing the Quality Chasm: A New Health System for the 21st Century*. Washington, DC: The National Academies Press.

Interprofessional Education Collaborative (IPEC). 2022. *Faculty Development Institutes*. https://www.ipecollaborative.org/institute.

Iobst, William F., Johnathan Sherbino, Olle Ten Cate, Denyse L. Richardson, Deepak Dath, Susan R. Swing, Peter Harris, et al. 2010. "Competency-Based Medical Education in Postgraduate Medical Education." *Medical Teacher*, *32*(8): 651–656. https://doi.org/10.3109/0142159X.2010.500709.

Israel, Emma, and Jeanne Batalova. 2021. "International Students in the United States." *Migration Information Source*, January 14, 2021. https://www.migrationpolicy.org/article/international-students-united-states-2020.

Jackson, Jason, Spencer Lin, and Marcelo Sávio. 2021. "The Edge Computing Advantage: Industrial Companies Unlock Efficiencies and Data-Rich Insights." *Research Insights*. Armack, NY: IBM Corporation. https://www.ibm.com/downloads/cas/Y7RA6X93.

Jackson, Sheryl. 2019. "Recruiters Tackle the Downturn in International Student Enrollment." *Insight into Diversity*, February 11, 2019. https://www.insightintodiversity.com/recruiters-tackle-the-downturn-in-international-student-enrollment/.

Jauregui, Joshua, Bjorn Watsjold, Laura Welsh, and Jonathan S. Ilgen. 2019. "Generational 'Othering': The Myth of the Millennial Learner." *Medical Education*, *54*(1): 60–65. https://doi.org/10.1111/medu.13795.

Jha, Vikram, Michelle McLean, Trevor Gibbs, and John Sandars. 2015. "Medical Professionalism across Cultures: A Challenge for Medicine and Medical Education." *Medical Teacher*, *37*(1): 74–80. https://doi.org/10.3109/0142159X.2014.920492.

Johnson, Daniel M. 2019. "Student Demographics: The Coming Changes and Challenges for Higher Education." In *The Uncertain Future of American Public Higher Education*, edited by Daniel M. Johnson, 141–156. Cham, Switzerland: Palgrave Macmillan. https://link.springer.com/chapter/10.1007/978-3-030-01794-1_10.

Jonas, Bruce S., Qiuping Gu, and Juan Albertorio-Diaz. 2013. "Psychotropic Medication Use among Adolescents: United States, 2005–2010." *National Center for Health Statistics Data Brief*, *135*: 1–8.

Jordan, Jaime, Daena Watcha, Courtney Cassella, Amy H. Kaji, and Shefali Trivedi. 2019. "Impact of a Mentorship Program on Medical Student Burnout. "*AEM Education and Training*, *3*(3): 218–225. https://doi.org/10.1002/aet2.10354.

Katoue, Maram Gamal, and Terry L. Schwinghammer. 2020. "Competency-Based Education in Pharmacy: A Review of Its Development, Applications, and Challenges." *Journal of Evaluation in Clinical Practice*, *26:* 1114–1123. https://doi.org/10.1111/jep.13362.

Kearney, Melissa S., and Phillip Levine. 2021. "Will Births in the US Rebound? Probably Not." Brookings Institution "Up Front" blog post, May 24, 2021. https://www.brookings.edu/blog/up-front/2021/05/24/will-births-in-the-us-reboundprobably-not/.

Keeling, Richard P. 2004. *Learning Reconsidered: A Campus-Wide Focus on the Student Experience*. Washington, DC: National Association of Student Personnel Administrators, American College Personnel Association.

Kelderman, Eric. 2021. "Making College More Affordable." In *Recruiting and Retaining Students in a Challenging Market*, edited by Kelly Field, Eric Kelderman, Katherine Mangan, and Brian O'Leary, 17–24. The Chronicle of Higher Education. https://store.chronicle.com/products/recruiting-and-retaining-students-in-a-challenging-market.

Kent, Julia D., and Maureen Terese McCarthy. 2016. *Holistic Review in Graduate Admissions: A Report from the Council of Graduate Schools*. Washington, DC: Council of Graduate Schools.

Killam, Wendy K., and Suzanne Degges-White. 2017. "Introduction to Student Affairs and Student Development Issues." In *College Student Development: Applying Theory to Practice on the Diverse Campus*, edited by Wendy K. Killam and Suzanne Degges-White, 1–12. Springer Publishing Company.

Killen, Roy. 2000. "Outcomes-Based Education: Principles and Possibilities." Unpublished manuscript, University of Newcastle, Faculty of Education. https://academic.payap.ac.th/pyu/uploads/userfiles/file/KM/2558/1_-2-Killen_paper_good-kena-baca1.pdf.

King, Heather B., James Battles, David P. Baker, Alexander Alonso, Eduardo Salas, John Webster, Lauren Toomey, and Mary Salisbury. 2008. "TeamSTEPPS™: Team Strategies and Tools to Enhance Performance and Patient Safety." In *Advances in Patient Safety: New Directions and Alternative Approaches,* edited by Kerm Henriksen, James B. Battles, Margaret A. Keyes, and Mary L. Grady, 5–20. Rockville, MD: Agency for Healthcare Research and Quality. https://www.ncbi.nlm.nih.gov/books/NBK43686/.

Kohn, Linda T., Janet Corrigan, and Molla S. Donaldson. 2000. *To Err Is Human: Building a Safer Health System*. Washington DC: National Academy Press.

Kolb, David A., Richard E. Boyatzis, and Charalampos Mainemelis. 2014. "Experiential Learning Theory: Previous Research and New Directions." In *Perspectives on Thinking, Learning, and Cognitive Styles*, edited by Robert J. Sternberg and Li-Fang Zhang, 227–248. New York: Routledge. https://doi.org/10.4324/9781410605986.

Kowarski, Ilana. 2020. "Are Medical School and Becoming a Doctor Worth It?" *U.S. News and World Report: Education*, July 16, 2020. https://www.usnews.com/education/best-graduate-schools/top-medical-schools/articles/how-to-decide-if-going-to-medical-school-and-being-a-doctor-is-worth-it.

Kristina, Susi Ari, and Yosef Wijoyo. 2019. "Assessment of Pharmacy Students' Clinical Skills Using Objective Structured Clinical Examination (OSCE): A Literature Review." *Systematic Review in Pharmacy*, *10*(1): 55–60. https://doi.org/10.5530/srp.2019.1.9.

Kron, Frederick W., Michael D. Fetters, Mark W. Scerbo, Casey B. White, Monica L. Lypson, Miguel A. Padilla, Gayle A. Gliva-McConvey, et al. 2017. "Using a Computer Simulation for Teaching Communication Skills: A Blinded Multisite Mixed Methods Randomized Controlled Trial." *Patient Education and Counseling*, *100*(4): 748–759. https://doi.org/10.1016/j.pec.2016.10.024.

Kubaryk, Lindsey. 2020a. "5 Forces Shaping Generation Z Present Opportunities and Major Challenges for Student Affairs." EAB, February 11, 2020. https://eab.com/insights/expert-insight/student-affairs/student-affairs-implications-as-gen-z-goes-to-college/.

Kubaryk, Lindsey. 2020b. "How Gen Z's Intensifying Demand for Mental Health Care Affects Campus Resources." EAB, March 4, 2020. https://eab.com/insights/expert-insight/student-affairs/gen-z-mental-health/.

Kupperschmidt, Betty R. 2000. "Multigeneration Employees: Strategies for Effective Management." *The Health Care Manager*, *19*(1): 65–76. https://doi.org/10.1097/00126450-200019010-00011.

Lammert, Catherine, and Andrea Malek Ash. 2022. "'So, When Do I Begin?' Critical Incidents of Successes (Plus a Few Mishaps) in Boomers' Mentorship of Millennials." In *The Changing Faces of Higher Education: From Boomers to Millennials*, edited by Mitchell B. Mackinem, Lacey J. Ritter, and Anisah Bagasra, 25–42. Wilmington, Delaware: Vernon Press.

Lebovitz, Lisa, and Mike Rudolph. 2020. "Update on Pharmacist Workforce Data and Thoughts on How to Manage the Oversupply." *American Journal of Pharmaceutical Education*, *84*(10). https://doi.org/10.5688/ajpe7889.

Lederman, Doug. 2021. "Detailing Last Fall's Online Enrollment Surge." *Inside Higher Ed*, September 16, 2021. https://www.insidehighered.com/news/2021/09/16/new-data-offer-sense-how-covid-expanded-online-learning.

Levine, Alaina G. 2017. "From Selfies to Selfless: Managing Multigenerational Teams." *Science Magazine*, September 14, 2017. https://www.science.org/content/article/selfies-selfless-managing-multigenerational-teams.

LeViness, Peter, Kim Gorman, Lynn Braun, Linda Koenig, and Carolyn Bershad. 2019. "The Association for University and College Counseling Center Directors: Annual Survey 2019." The Association for University and College Counseling Center Directors. https://www.aucccd.org/assets/documents/Survey/2019%20AUCCCD%20Survey-2020-05-31-PUBLIC.pdf.

Lewis, Lisa S., Lisa M. Rebeschi, and Ellie Hunt. 2022. "Nursing Education Practice Update 2022: Competency-Based Education in Nursing." *SAGE Open Nursing*, *8*, https://doi.org/10.1177/23779608221140774.

Lipson, Sarah Ketchen, Sara Abelson, Peter Ceglarek, Megan Phillips, and Daniel Eisenberg. 2019. "Investing in Student Mental Health: Opportunities and Benefits for College Leadership." Washington, DC: American Council on Education. https://www.acenet.edu/Documents/Investing-in-Student-Mental-Health.pdf.

Little, Meg M., Catherine A. St. Hill, Kenric B. Ware, Michael T. Swanoski, Scott A. Chapman, M. Nawal Lutfiyya, and Frank B. Cerra. 2017. "Team Science as Interprofessional Collaborative Research Practice: A Systematic Review of the Science of Team Science Literature." *Journal of Investigative Medicine*, *65*(1): 15–22. https://doi.org/10.1136/jim-2016-000216.

Livingston, G., and D. Cohn. 2010. "US Birth Rate Decline Linked to Recession. Pew Research Center Demographic Trends Report." https://www.pewresearch.org/social-trends/2010/04/06/us-birth-rate-decline-linked-to-recession/.

Lockwood, Penelope, Christian H. Jordan, and Ziva Kunda. 2002. "Motivation by Positive or Negative Role Models: Regulatory Focus Determines Who Will Best inspire Us." *Journal of Personality and Social Psychology*, *83*(4): 854–864. https://doi.org/10.1037//0022-3514.83.4.854.

Long, Dallas. 2012. "The Foundations of Student Affairs: A Guide to the Profession." In *Environments for Student Growth and Development: Librarians and Student Affairs in Collaboration*, edited by Lisa Janicke Hinchliffe and Melissa Autumn Wong, 1–39. Chicago: Association of College and Research Libraries. https://ir.library.illinoisstate.edu/cgi/viewcontent.cgi?article=1028&context=fpml.

Looker, Peter. 2020. "The Role of AR and VR in Learning and Assessment." EON Reality, June 1, 2020. https://eonreality.com/role-of-ar-and-vr-in-learning-and-assessment/.

Louie, Alan K., John H. Coverdale, Richard Balon, Eugene V. Beresin, Adam Brenner, Anthony P. S. Guerrero, and Laura Weiss. 2018. "Enhancing Empathy: A Role for Virtual Reality?" *Academic Psychiatry*, *42*(6): 747–752. https://doi.org/10.1007/s40596-018-0995-2.

Lurie, Howard, and Richard Garrett. 2017. "Deconstructing Competency-Based Education: An Assessment of Institutional Activity, Goals, and Challenges in Higher Education." *The Journal of Competency-Based Education*, *2*(3): e01047. https://doi.org/10.1002/cbe2.1047.

Ma, Gloria Yuet Kwan, and Winnie W. S. Mak. 2022. "Meta-Analysis of Studies on the Impact of Mobility Disability Simulation Programs on Attitudes toward People with Disabilities and Environmental In/accessibility." *PLoS One*, *17*(6): e0269357. https://doi.org/10.1371/journal.pone.0269357.

MacPhee, John, Kamla Modi, Sara Gorman, Nance Roy, Erica Riba, Diana Cusumano, John Dunkle, et al. 2021. "Strengthening Safety Nets: A Comprehensive Approach to Mental Health Promotion and Suicide Prevention for Colleges and Universities." National Academy of Medicine. https://nam.edu/a-comprehensive-approach-to-mental-health-promotion-and-suicide-prevention-for-colleges-and-universities-insights-from-the-jed-campus-program/.

Maerten-Rivera, Jaime L., Aleda M. H. Chen, Jill Augustine, Richard d'Assalenaux, Kelly C. Lee, Cameron C. Lindsey, Daniel R. Malcom, et al. 2020. "Co-Curriculum Implementation and Assessment in Accredited Doctor of Pharmacy Programs."

American Journal of Pharmaceutical Education, *84*(3): 7569. https://doi.org/10.5688/ajpe7569.

Maurer, Trent W. 2022. "Leveraging SoTL to Improve Teaching and Learning during the COVID-19 Pandemic," *International Journal for the Scholarship of Teaching and Learning*, *16*(1): Article 3. https://doi.org/10.20429/ijsotl.2022.160103.

McCarthy, Mary. 2016. "Experiential Learning Theory: From Theory to Practice." *Journal of Business & Economics Research*, *14*(3): 91–100. https://doi.org/10.19030/jber.v14i3.9749.

McClellan, George S., and Jeremy Stringer. 2016. *The Handbook of Student Affairs Administration*, fourth edition. San Francisco: Jossey-Bass.

McDonough, Sharon L. K., Erika L. Kleppinger, Amy R. Donaldson, and Kristen L. Helms. 2015. "Going 'High Stakes' with a Pharmacy OSCE: Lessons Learned in the Transition." *Currents in Pharmacy Teaching and Learning*, *7*(1): 4–11. https://doi.org/10.1016/j.cptl.2014.09.017.

McGaghie, William C., Saul B. Issenberg, Jeffrey H. Barsuk, and Diane B. Wayne. 2014. "A Critical Review of Simulation-based Mastery Learning with Translational Outcomes." *Medical Education*, *48*(4): 375–385. https://doi.org/10.1111/medu.12391.

McGuire, Lisa E., and Lay, Kathy A. 2020. "Reflective Pedagogy for Social Work Education: Integrating Classroom and Field for Competency-Based Education." *Journal of Social Work Education*, *56*(3): 519–532. https://doi.org/10.1080/10437797.2019.1661898.

McIntyre-Hite, Lisa. 2016. "A Delphi Study of Effective Practices for Developing Competency-Based Learning Models in Higher Education." *The Journal of Competency-Based Education*, *1*(4): 157–166. https://doi.org/10.1002/cbe2.1029.

McKeachie, Wilbert, and Marilla Svinicki. 2014. *McKeachie's Teaching Tips: Strategies, Research, and Theory for College and University Teachers*. Belmont, CA: Wadsworth Cengage Learning.

Meeks, Lisa M., Ben Case, Erene Stergiopoulos, Brianna K. Evans, and Kristina H. Petersen. 2021. "Structural Barriers to Student Disability Disclosure in US-Allopathic Medical Schools." *Journal of Medical Education and Curricular Development*, *8*, https://doi.org/10.1177/23821205211018696.

Mellman, Lisa A., and Brian Paquette. 2012. "Academic and Career Counseling for Medical Students and the Complex Role of the Student Affairs Dean." *Academic Psychiatry*, *36*(3): 169. https://doi.org/10.1176/appi.ap.10020034.

Mental Health by the Numbers. n.d. "National Alliance on Mental Health." https://www.nami.org/mhstats.

Merton, Robert K. 1957. "Some Preliminaries to a Sociology of Medical Education." In *The Student Physician: Introductory Studies in the Sociology of Medical Education*, edited by Robert K. Merton, George G. Reader, and Patricia L. Kendall, 3–79. Cambridge: Harvard University Press. https://doi.org/10.4159/Harvard.9780674366831.c2.

Meyers, Steven A. 2011. "Do Your Students Care Whether You Care about Them?" *College Teaching*, *57*(4): 205–210. https://doi.org/10.1080/87567550903218620.

Microsoft. 2021. "Work Trend Index Annual Report." Accessed on March 16, 2022. https://www.microsoft.com/en-us/worklab/work-trend-index/.

Miller, Amy Chasteen, and Brooklyn Mills. 2019. "'If They Don't Care, I Don't Care': Millennial and Generation Z Students and the Impact of Faculty Caring." *Journal of the Scholarship of Teaching and Learning*, *19*(4): 78–89. https://doi.org/10.14434/josotl.v19i4.24167.

Miller, George E. 1990. "The Assessment of Clinical Skills/Competence/Performance." *Academic Medicine*, *65*(9): S63–S67. https://doi.org/10.1097/00001888-199009000-00045.

Milk, Chris. 2015. "Virtual Reality Is the Ultimate Empathy Machine." March 2015. Presentation at TED 2015, 10:16. https://www.ted.com/talks/chris_milk_how_virtual_reality_can_create_the_ultimate_empathy_machine?language=en.

Mintz, Steven, and Michael Patrick Rutter. 2016. "The Curricular and Co-Curricular: The Importance of What Takes Place outside the Classroom." *Inside Higher Ed*. https://www.insidehighered.com/blogs/higher-ed-gamma/curricular-and-co-curricular.

Mistry, Neel, and Paul Rooprai. 2020. "First, Do No Harm: Trust Is Paramount in Healthcare." *Healthy Debate*, June 9, 2020. https://healthydebate.ca/2020/06/topic/trust-is-paramount-in-healthcare/.

Mohr, Kathleen A., and Eric S Mohr. 2017. "Understanding Generation Z Students to Promote a Contemporary Learning Environment." *Journal on Empowering Teaching Excellence*, *1*(1): Article 9. https://doi.org/10.15142/T3M05T.

Moore, Jill, Marcee Everly, and Renee Bauer. 2016. "Multigenerational Challenges: Team-Building for Positive Clinical Workforce Outcomes." *OJIN: The Online Journal of Issues in Nursing*, *21*(2): Manuscript 3. https://doi.org/10.3912/OJIN.Vol21No02Man03.

Morris, Devin B., Philip A. Gruppuso, Heather A. McGee, Anarina L. Murillo, Atul Grover, and Eli Y. Adashi. 2021. "Diversity of the National Medical Student Body – Four Decades of Inequities." *The New England Journal of Medicine*, *384*(17): 1661–1668. https://doi.org/10.1056/NEJMsr2028487.

Moseley, Lindsey E., Lauren McConnell, Kimberly B. Garza, and Channing R. Ford. 2021. "Exploring the Evolution of Professional Identity Formation in Health Professions Education." In *Cultivating Professional Identity Formation in the Health Sciences*, edited by Channing R. Ford, Lindsey E. Moseley, and Kimberly B. Garza. *New Directions of Teaching and Learning*, *2021*(169): 11–27. https://doi.org/10.1002/tl.20464.

Mundell, Chris. 2022. "Doing No Harm: One Practitioner's Journey towards Trauma-Informed Practice." In "Trauma-Informed Practice in Student Affairs: Multidimensional Considerations for Care, Healing, and Wellbeing," edited by Tricia R. Shalka, and Wilson K. Okello. *New Directions for Student Services*, *2022*(177): 17–25. https://doi.org/10.1002/ss.20411.

Mylrea, Martina F., Tarun Sen Gupta, and Beverley D. Glass. 2015. "Professionalization in Pharmacy Education as a Matter of Identity." *American Journal of Pharmaceutical Education*, *79*(9): Article 142. https://doi.org/10.5688/ajpe799142.

Mylrea, Martina F., Tarun Sen Gupta, and Beverley D. Glass. 2017. "Validation of a Motivation Survey Tool for Pharmacy Students: Exploring a Link to Professional

Identity Development." *Currents in Pharmacy Teaching and Learning*, *9*(5): 763–769. https://doi.org/10.1016/j.cptl.2017.05.014.

Mylrea, Martina F., Tarun Sen Gupta, and Beverley D. Glass. 2019. "Design and Evaluation of a Professional Identity Development Program for Pharmacy Students." *American Journal of Pharmaceutical Education*, *83*(6): 6842. https://doi.org/10.5688/ajpe6842.

NASPA: Student Affairs Administrators in Higher Education. March 2022. *The Compass Report: Charting the Future of Student Affairs.*

NASPA: Student Affairs Administrators in Higher Education. n.d. "About Student Affairs." https://naspa.org/about/about-student-affairs/about-student-affairs.

National Academies of Sciences, Engineering, and Medicine. 2019. *Taking Action against Clinician Burnout: A Systems Approach to Professional Well-Being*. Washington, DC: The National Academies Press.

National Center for Education Statistics. 2018. "Table 311.10. Number and Percentage Distribution of Students Enrolled in Postsecondary Institutions, by Level, Disability Status, and Selected Student Characteristics: 2015–16 [Data table]." In *Digest of Education Statistics*. U.S. Department of Education, Institute of Education Sciences. https://nces.ed.gov/programs/digest/d20/tables/dt20_311.10.asp.

National Center for Education Statistics. 2020a. "Table 302.85. Among Adults 18 years old and over who Reported all Fall Attendance Plans for at Least One Adult in Their Household had been Canceled, Percentage Reporting on Reasons for Changes in Plans, by Level of Postsecondary Education Planned and Selected Respondent Characteristics [Data table]." In *Digest of Education Statistics*. U.S. Department of Education, Institute of Education Sciences. https://nces.ed.gov/programs/digest/d20/tables/dt20_302.85.asp

National Center for Education Statistics. 2020b. "Table 303.40. Total Fall Enrollment in Degree Granting Post-Secondary Institutions, By Attendance Status, Sex, and Age of Student: Selected Years, 1970 through 2029 [Data table]." In *Digest of Education Statistics*. U.S. Department of Education, Institute of Education Sciences. https://nces.ed.gov/programs/digest/d20/tables/dt20_303.40.asp.

National Center for Education Statistics. 2021. "Table 302.85. Among Adults 18 years old and over who Reported all Fall Attendance Plans for at Least One Adult in Their Household had been Canceled, Percentage Reporting on Reasons for Changes in Plans, by Selected Respondent Characteristics [Data table]." In *Digest of Education Statistics*. U.S. Department of Education, Institute of Education Sciences. https://nces.ed.gov/programs/digest/d21/tables/dt21_302.85.asp.

National Center for Education Statistics. 2022. "Characteristics of PostSecondary Students." *Condition of Education*. U.S. Department of Education, Institute of Education Sciences. https://nces.ed.gov/programs/coe/indicator/csb/postsecondary-students.

National Center for Higher Education Management Systems. n.d. "College-Going Rates of High School Graduates – Directly from High School." Accessed February 28, 2022. http://www.higheredinfo.org/dbrowser/?year=2002&level=nation&mode=data&state=&submeasure=63#/-1/.

National Center for Interprofessional Practice and Education. n.d. "Assessment and Evaluation." Accessed December 11, 2022. https://nexusipe.org/advancing/assessment-evaluation.

National Student Clearinghouse Research Center. 2022a. "Current Term Enrollment Estimates." National Student Clearinghouse, Accessed May 26, 2022. https://nscresearchcenter.org/current-term-enrollment-estimates/.

National Student Clearinghouse Research Center. 2022b. "Stay Informed with the Latest Enrollment Information: National Student Clearinghouse Research Center's Regular Updates on Higher Education Enrollment." National Student Clearinghouse, October 20, 2022. https://nscresearchcenter.org/stay-informed/.

Newble, David I., and David B. Swanson. 1998. "Psychometric Characteristics of the Objective Structured Clinical Examination." *Medical Education, 22*(4): 325–334. https://doi.org/10.1111/j.1365-2923.1988.tb00761.x.

Newport, Cal. 2018. *DEEP WORK: Rules for Focused Success in a Distracted World.* New York: Grand Central Publishing.

Noble, Christy, Leigh McKauge, and Alexandria Clavarino. 2019. "Pharmacy Student Professional Identity Formation: A Scoping Review." *Integrated Pharmacy Research & Practice, 8:* 15–34. https://doi.org/10.2147/IPRP.S162799.

North American Moving Services. 2021. "Where Are Americans Moving in 2021?" Accessed December 11, 2022. https://www.northamerican.com/migration-map.

North Arizona University Teaching Academy. 2016. "Using Interprofessional Education in Your Multigenerational Classroom." Teaching with Fire Blog, February 26, 2016, https://in.nau.edu/teaching-academy/using-interprofessional-education-in-your-multigenerational-classroom/.

Novilla, M. Lelinneth B., Victor B. A. Moxley, Carl L. Hanson, Alisha H. Rédelas, Jeffrey Glenn, Paola G. Donoso Naranjo, Jenna M. S. Smith, Lynneth Kirsten B. Novilla, Sarah Stone, and Rachel Lafitaga. 2023. "COVID-19 and Psychosocial Well-Being: Did COVID-19 Worsen U.S. Frontline Healthcare Workers' Burnout, Anxiety, and Depression?" *International Journal of Environmental Research and Public Health, 20*: 4414. https://doi.org/10.3390/ijerph20054414.

Odell, Sandra J. 1990. *Mentor Teacher Program. What Research Says to the Teacher.* Washington, DC: National Education Association. https://files.eric.ed.gov/fulltext/ED323185.pdf.

One Million Degrees. 2022. Accessed December 15, 2022. https://onemilliondegrees.org/.

Pan, Xueni, Mel Slater, Alejandro Beacco, Xavi Navarro, Anna I. Bellido Rivas, David Swapp, Joanna Hale, et al. 2016. "The Responses of Medical General Practitioners to Unreasonable Patient Demand for Antibiotics – A Study of Medical Ethics Using Immersive Virtual Reality." *PloS one, 11*(2): e0146837. https://doi.org/10.1371/journal.pone.0146837.

Parker, Kim, and Juliana Horowitz. 2022. "Majority of Workers Who Quit a Job in 2021 Cite Low Pay, No Opportunities for Advancement, Feeling Disrespected." Pew Research Center, March 9, 2022. https://www.pewresearch.org/fact-tank/2022/03/09/majority-of-workers-who-quit-a-job-in-2021-cite-low-pay-no-opportunities-for-advancement-feeling-disrespected/.

Parker, Kim, and Ruth Igielnik. 2020. "On the Cusp of Adulthood and Facing an Uncertain Future: What We Know about Gen Z So Far." Pew Research Center, May 14, 2020. https://www.pewresearch.org/social-trends/2020/05/14/on-the-cusp-of-adulthood-and-facing-an-uncertain-future-what-we-know-about-gen-z-so-far-2/.

Patch, Will. 2021. "Class of Fall 2022 Senior Survey." *NICHE*, October 25, 2021. https://www.niche.com/about/enrollment-insights/class-of-2022-fall-senior-survey/

Paul, Dereck W. 2019. "Medical Training in the Maelstrom: The Call to Physician Advocacy and Activism in Turbulent Times." *Academic Medicine*, *94*(8): 1071–1073. https://doi.org/10.1097/ACM.0000000000002765.

Paullett, Karen, Diana Behling, and Robert Behling. 2020. "The Role of Higher Education Institutions in Reskilling the Workforce." *Issues in Information Systems*, *21*(1): 49–54. https://doi.org/10.48009/1_iis_2020_49–54.

Pedrelli, Paola, Maren Nyer, Albert Yeung, Courtney Zulauf, and Timothy Wilens. 2015. "College Students: Mental Health Problems and Treatment Considerations." *Academic Psychiatry*, *39*(5): 503–11. https://doi.org/10.1007/s40596-014-0205-9.

Perez, Rosemary J. 2016. "A Conceptual Model of Professional Socialization within Student Affairs Graduate Preparation Programs." *Journal for the Study of Postsecondary and Tertiary Education*, *1*: 35–52. https://doi.org/10.28945/2344.

Peritz, Aki. 2022. "A.I. Is Making It Easier than Ever for Students to Cheat." *Slate*, September 6, 2022. https://slate.com/technology/2022/09/ai-students-writing-cheating-sudowrite.html.

Percheski, Christine, and Rachel Kimbro. 2014. "How Did the Great Recession Affect Fertility." *Focus*, *30*(2): 26–30.

Perkins, Kelli A., and Glenn Herring. 2021. "Generational Perspective and Influence within Student Affairs Workplaces." In "Supervision in Student Affairs: Approaches and Tensions in Today's Workplaces," edited by Tiffany J. Davis and Brittany M. Williams. *New Directions for Student Services*, *2021*(175): 73–82. https://doi.org/10.1002/ss.20398.

Perna, Mark C. 2021. "Why Skill and Career Advancement Are the Way to Gen-Z's Heart." *Forbes*, March 2, 2021. https://www.forbes.com/sites/markcperna/2021/03/02/why-skill-and-career-advancement-are-the-way-to-gen-zs-heart/?sh=42b1561f22b5.

Pew Research Center. 2014. *Millennials in adulthood*. http://www.pewsocialtrends.org/2014/03/07/millennials-in-adulthood/.

Pew Research Center. 2015. "The Whys and Hows of Generations Research." Pew Research Center – *U.S. Politics & Policy*, September 3, 2015. https://www.pewresearch.org/politics/2015/09/03/the-whys-and-hows-of-generations-research/.

Pew Research Center. 2019. "Defining Generations: Where Millennials End and Generation Z Begins." Pew Research Center, January 17, 2019. https://www.pewresearch.org/fact-tank/2019/01/17/where-millennials-end-and-generation-z-begins/.

Pew Research Center. 2020. "On the Cusp of Adulthood and Facing an Uncertain Future: What We Know about Gen Z So Far." Pew Research Center – *Social*

Trends, May 14, 2020. https://www.pewresearch.org/social-trends/2020/05/14/on-the-cusp-of-adulthood-and-facing-an-uncertain-future-what-we-know-about-gen-z-so-far-2/.

Pfeifer, Jacob, Andrew Egger, Molly Hughes, Lauren Tondl, Robin High, and Kari L. Nelson. 2022. "An Investigation of Stress and Anxiety among Health Professions Students in the Early Stages of the COVID-19 Pandemic." *Journal of Interprofessional Education & Practice*, *28*, 100531. https://doi.org/10.1016/j.xjep.2022.100531.

Phillips, Kevin E. 2019. Managing Millennials: The Ultimate Handbook for Productivity, Profitability, and Professionalism. New York: Routledge. https://doi.org/10.4324/9781351054942.

Pizzinelli, Carlo, and Ippei Shibata. 2022. "Why Jobs Are Plentiful While Workers Are Scarce." IMF Blog, January 19, 2022. https://www.imf.org/en/Blogs/Articles/2022/01/19/why-jobs-are-plentiful-while-workers-are-scarce.

Plochocki, Jeffrey H. 2019. "Several Ways Generation Z May Shape the Medical School Landscape." *Journal of Medical Education and Curricular Development*, *6*, https://doi.org/10.1177/2382120519884325.

Plunkett, Anthony D. 2014. "A's for Everyone: The Effects of Student Consumerism in the Postsecondary Classroom." *The Qualitative Report*, *19*(12): 1–3. https://doi.org/10.46743/2160-3715/2014.1258.

Potter, Michael K., and Erika D. H. Kustra. 2011. "The Relationship between Scholarly Teaching and SoTL: Models, Distinctions, and Clarifications," *International Journal for the Scholarship of Teaching and Learning*, *5*(1): Article 23. https://doi.org/10.20429/ijsotl.2011.050123.

Pottle, Jack. 2019. "Virtual Reality and the Transformation of Medical Education." *Future Healthcare Journal*, *6*(3): 181–185. https://doi.org/10.7861/fhj.2019-0036.

Povejsil, Elise. 2021. "How Colleges Can Reinvent the Enrollment Funnel." *Collegis Education*. March 18, 2021. https://collegiseducation.com/news/marketing/reinventing-the-enrollment-funnel/.

Prater, M. Renee. 2020. "Teaching Millennials and Generation Z: New Opportunities in Undergraduate Medical Education." In *Handbook of Research on the Efficacy of Training Programs and Systems in Medical Education*, edited by Ruth Gotian, Yoon Kang, and Joseph Safdieh, 72–91. Hershey, PA: IGI Global. https://doi.org/10.4018/978-1-7998-1468-9.ch004.

Project Quest. 2021. Accessed December 15, 2022. https://questsa.org/.

Puentedura, Ruben R. 2014. Building Transformation: An Introduction to the SAMR Model (blog). http://www.hippasus.com/rrpweblog/archives/2014/08/22/BuildingTransformation_AnIntroductionToSAMR.pdf.

Rainwater, Terese S. M. 2015. "Teaching and Learning in Competency-Based Education Courses and Programs: Faculty and Student Perspectives." *The Journal of Competency-Based Education*, *1*(1): 42–47. https://doi.org/10.1002/cbe2.1008.

Reed, Darcy A., Tait D. Shanafelt, Daniel W. Satele, David V. Power, Anne Eacker, William Harper, Christine Moutier, et al. 2011. "Relationship of Pass/Fail Grading and Curriculum Structure with Well-Being among Preclinical Medical Students: A

Multi-Institutional Study." *Academic Medicine*, *86*(11): 1367–1373. https://doi.org/10.1097/ACM.0b013e3182305d81.

Reeves, Richard V., and Ember Smith. 2021. "The Male College Crisis in Not Just Enrollment, but Completion." Brookings, October 8, 2021. https://www.brookings.edu/blog/up-front/2021/10/08/the-male-college-crisis-is-not-just-in-enrollment-but-completion/.

Reeves, Scott, Merrick Zwarenstein, Joanne Goldman, Hugh Barr, Della Freeth, Marilyn Hammick, and Ivan Koppel. 2008. "Interprofessional Education: Effects on Professional Practice and Health Care Outcomes." *The Cochrane Database of Systematic Reviews*, (1): CD002213. https://doi.org/10.1002/14651858.CD002213.pub2.

Reeves, Scott, Simon Fletcher, Hugh Barr, Ivan Birch, Sylvain Boet, Nigel Davies, Angus McFadyen, Josette Rivera, and Simon Kitto. 2016. "A BEME Systematic Review of the Effects of Interprofessional Education: BEME Guide No. 39." *Medical Teacher*, *38*(7): 656–668. https://doi.org/10.3109/0142159X.2016.1173663.

Regehr, Glenn. 2020. "'Kids These Days': Reconsidering Our Conversations about Millennial Learners." *Medical Education*, *54*(1): 10–12. https://doi.org/10.1111/medu.14002.

Rhyneer Madeleine. 2021. "How to Effectively Reach Gen Z in 2022." *EAB*, June 1, 2021. https://eab.com/insights/blogs/enrollment/effectively-reach-gen-z/.

Rickes, Persis C. 2016. "Generations in Flux: How Gen Z Will Continue to Transform Higher Education Space." *Planning for Higher Education*, *44*(4): 21–45.

Roberts, Darby. 2019. "Extracurricular vs. Co-curricular." *Student Affairs Planning Assessment and Research* (blog), Texas A&M, January 2, 2019. https://studentlifestudies.tamu.edu/extracurricular-vs-co-curricular/.

Robertson, Noah. 2021. "Men Are Missing from College Campuses: What's Being Done to Bring Them Back?" *Christian Science Monitor*, November 9. 2021, 9. https://www.csmonitor.com/USA/Education/2021/1109/Men-are-missing-from-college-campuses-What-s-being-done-to-bring-them-back.

Rodger, Sylvia, Steven J. Hoffman, and World Health Organization Study Group on Interprofessional Education and Collaborative Practice. 2010. "Where in the World Is Interprofessional Education? A Global Environmental Scan." *Journal of Interprofessional Care*, *24*(5): 479–491. https://doi.org/10.3109/13561821003721329.

Rosseter, Robert. October 2022. "Nursing Faculty Shortage Fact Sheet." American Association of Colleges of Nursing. https://www.aacnnursing.org/Portals/0/PDFs/Fact-Sheets/Faculty-Shortage-Factsheet.pdf.

Schenarts, Paul J. 2020. "Now Arriving: Surgical Trainees from Generation Z." *Journal of Surgical Education*, *77*(2): 246–253. https://doi.org/10.1016/j.jsurg.2019.09.004.

Schoeb, Dominik S., Jan Schwarz, Simon Hein, Daniel Schlager, Philippe F. Pohlmann, Alexander Frankenschmidt, Christian Gratzke, and Arkadiusz Miernik. 2020. "Mixed Reality for Teaching Catheter Placement to Medical

Students: A Randomized Single-Blinded, Prospective Trial." *BMC Medical Education*, *20*(1): 510. https://doi.org/10.1186/s12909-020-02450-5.

Schroeder, Ray. 2021. "A Second Demographic Cliff Adds to Urgency for Change." Inside Higher Ed, May 19, 2021. https://www.insidehighered.com/digital-learning/blogs/online-trending-now/second-demographic-cliff-adds-urgency-change.

Schroth, Holly. 2019. "Are You Ready for Gen Z in the Workplace?" *California Management Review*, *61*(3): 5–18. https://doi.org/10.1177/0008125619841006.

Schuh, John H., Susan R. Jones, and Vasti Torres. 2017. *Student Services: A Handbook for the Profession*, sixth edition. San Francisco: Jossey-Bass.

Seemiller, Corey, and Meghan Grace. 2016. *Generation Z Goes to College*. San Francisco: Jossey-Bass.

Seemiller, Corey, and Meghan Grace. 2017a. "Generation Z: Educating and Engaging the Next Generation of Students." *About Campus*, *22*(3): 21–26. https://doi.org/10.1002/abc.21293.

Seemiller, Corey, and Meghan Grace. 2017b. *Generation Z Leads: A Guide for Developing the Leadership Capacity of Generation Z Students*. Independently Published.

Seemiller, Corey, and Meghan Grace. 2019a. *Generation Z: A Century in the Making*. New York: Routledge.

Seemiller, Corey, and Meghan Grace. 2019b. *Generation Z Learns: A Guide for Engaging Generation Z Students in Meaningful Learning*. Independently Published.

Selingo, Jeffrey J. 2021. *The Future of Gen Z: How COVID-19 Will Shape Students and Higher Education in the Next Decade*. The Chronicle of Higher Education. https://store.chronicle.com/products/the-future-of-gen-z.

Shatto, Bobbi, and Kelly Erwin. 2016. "Moving on from Millennials: Preparing for Generation Z." *The Journal of Continuing Education in Nursing*, *47*(6): 253–254. https://doi.org/10.3928/00220124-20160518-05.

Shatto, Bobbi, and Kelly Erwin. 2017. "Teaching Millennials and Generation Z: Bridging the Generational Divide." *Creative Nursing*, *23*(1): 24–28. https://doi.org/10.1891/1078-4535.23.1.24.

Shiralkar Malan T., Toi B. Harris, Florence F. Eddins-Folensbee, and John H. Cloverdale. 2013. "A Systematic Review of Stress Management Programs for Medical Students." *Academic Psychiatry*, *37*: 158–164. https://doi.org/10.1176/appi.ap.12010003.

Shorey, Shefaly, Valerie Chan, Priyadharshni Rajendran, and Emily Ang. 2021. "Learning Styles, Preferences, and Needs of Generation Z Healthcare Students: A Scoping Review." *Nurse Education in Practice*, *57*: 103247. https://doi.org/10.1016/j.nepr.2021.103247.

Silver, Ivan I., and Karen Leslie. 2017. "Faculty Development for Continuing Interprofessional Education and Collaborative Practice." *Journal of Continuing Education in the Health Professions*, *37*(4): 262–267. https://doi.org/10.1097/CEH.0000000000000178.

Silverman, Arielle Michal. 2015. "The Perils of Playing Blind: Problems with Blindness Simulation and a Better Way to Teach about Blindness." *Journal of Blindness and Innovation Research*, *5*(2).

Sistermans, Ilse Johanna. 2020. "Integrating Competency-Based Education with a Case-Based or Problem-Based Learning Approach in Online Health Sciences. *Asia Pacific Education Review*, *21*: 683–696. https://doi.org/10.1007/s12564-020-09658-6.

Slate, John R., Kimberly Nichols LaPrairie, Don P. Schulte, and Anthony J. Onwuegbuzie. 2011. "Views of Effective College Faculty: A Mixed Analysis." *Assessment & Evaluation in Higher Education*, *36*(3): 331–346. https://doi.org/10.1080/02602930903428684.

Small, Gary W., Jooyeon Lee, Aaron Kaufman, Jason Jalil, Prabha Siddarth, Himaja Gaddipati, Teena D. Moody, and Susan Y. Bookheimer. 2020. "Brain Health Consequences of Digital Technology Use." *Dialogues in Clinical Neuroscience*, *22*(2): 179–187. https://doi.org/10.31887/DCNS.2020.22.2/gsmall.

Smith, Cynthia D., Celynne Balatbat, Susan Corbridge, Anna Legried Dopp, Jessica Fried, Ron Harter, Seth Landefeld, et al. 2018. "Implementing Optimal Team-based Care to Reduce Clinician Burnout." *NAM Perspectives.* Discussion Paper, National Academy of Medicine, Washington, DC. https://doi.org/10.31478/201809c.

Soria, Krista M., and Bonnie Horgos. 2021. "Factors Associated with College Students' Mental Health during the COVID-19 Pandemic." *Journal of College Student Development*, *62*(2): 236–42. https://doi.org/10.1353/csd.2021.0024.

Sorcinelli, Mary Deane. 2002. "Ten Principles of Good Practice in Creating and Sustaining Teaching and Learning Centers." In *A Guide to Faculty Development: Practical Advice, Examples, and Resources*, edited by Kay Herr Gillespie, 9–23.

Srinivasan, Vasanthi. 2012. "Multi Generations in the Workforce: Building Collaboration." *IIMB Management Review*, *24*(1): 48–66. https://doi.org/10.1016/j.iimb.2012.01.004.

Statista. 2022. *Global Digital Population as of April 2022.* https://www.statista.com/statistics/617136/digital-population-worldwide/.

Steele Flippin, Candace. 2017. *Generation Z in the Workplace: Helping the Newest Generation in the Workforce Build Successful Working Relationships and Career Paths*. United States: Independently Published.

Stoehr, Fabian, Lukas Müller, Adrian Brady, Antoni Trilla, Aline Mähringer-Kunz, Felix Hahn, Christoph Düber, et al. 2021. "How COVID-19 Kick-Started Online Learning in Medical Education—The DigiMed Study." *PloS One*, *16*(9): e0257394. https://doi.org/10.1371/journal.pone.0257394.

Stoet, Gijsbert, and David C. Geary. 2020. "Gender Differences in the Pathways to Higher Education." *Proceedings of the National Academy of Sciences*, *117*(25): 14703–14706. https://doi.org/10.1073/pnas.2002861117.

Strauss, William, and Neil Howe. 1991. *Generations: The History of America's Future, 1584 to 2069.* New York: William Morrow & Co.

Substance Abuse and Mental Health Services Administration. 2020. "Key Substance Use and Mental Health Indicators in the United States: Results from the 2020 National Survey on Drug Use and Health." Rockville, MD: Center for Behavioral Health Statistics and Quality, Substance Abuse and Mental Health Services Administration. https://www.samhsa.gov/data/sites/default/files/reports/

rpt35325/NSDUHFFRPDFWHTMLFiles2020/2020NSDUHFFR1PDFW102121.pdf.

Sukhera, Javeed, and Chris Watling. 2018. "A Framework for Integrating Implicit Bias Recognition into Health Professions Education." *Academic Medicine*, *93*(1): 35–40. https://doi.org/10.1097/acm.0000000000001819.

Swanzen, Rika. 2018. "Facing the Generation Chasm: The Parenting and Teaching of Generations Y and Z." *International Journal of Child, Youth, and Family Studies*, *9*(2): 125–150. https://doi.org/10.18357/ijcyfs92201818216.

Szymkowiak, Andrzej, Boban Melovic, Marina Dabic, Kishokanth Jeganathan, and Gagandeep Singh Kundi. 2021. "Information Technology and Gen Z: The Role of Teachers, The Internet, and Technology in the Education of Young People." *Technology in Society*, 65, 101565. https://doi.org/10.1016/j.techsoc.2021.101565.

Taylor, Kevin M. G., and Geoffrey Harding. 2007. "The Pharmacy Degree: The Student Experience of Professional Training." *Pharmacy Education*, *7*(1): 83–88. https://pharmacyeducation.fip.org/pharmacyeducation/article/view/238.

Taylor, Melissa Kempf. 2018. "Xennials: A Microgeneration in the Workplace." *Industrial and Commercial Training*, *50*(3): 136–147. https://doi.org/10.1108/ICT-08-2017-0065.

Texas Center for Nursing Workforce Studies. 2022. "Professional Nursing Education Reports." *Texas Health and Human Services*. https://www.dshs.texas.gov/chs/cnws/Nursing-Education-Reports.aspx

The California State University. n.d. "How We're Implementing Change." https://www.calstate.edu/csu-system/why-the-csu-matters/graduation-initiative-2025/How-Were-Implementing-Change.

The Chronicle of Higher Education. Webinar accessed February 17, 2022. "The Demographic Cliff: Surviving Enrollment Challenges."

The Healthy Minds Study. 2021. "The Health Minds Study: 2021 Winter/Spring Data Report." https://healthymindsnetwork.org/wp-content/uploads/2022/01/HMS_nationalwinter2021_-update1.5.21.pdf.

The Ohio State University College of Nursing. 2023. "Office of Student Affairs and Success." https://nursing.osu.edu/offices-and-initiatives/office-student-affairs-and-success#:~:text=The%20Office%20of%20Student%20Affairs,records%20management%20and%20program%20compliance.

Trede, Franziska, Rob Macklin, and Donna Bridges. 2012. "Professional Identity Development: A Review of Higher Education Literature." *Studies in Higher Education*, *37*(3): 365–384. https://doi.org/10.1080/03075079.2010.521237.

Tuomikoski, Anna-Maria, Heidi Ruotsalainen, Kristina Mikkonen, and Maria Kääriäinen. 2020. "Nurses' Experiences of Their Competence at mentoring nursing students during Clinical Practice: A Systematic Review of Qualitative Studies." *Nurse Education Today*, *85*, 104258. https://doi.org/10.1016/j.nedt.2019.104258.

Tyton Partners, and Babson Survey Research Group. 2019. "Driving toward a Degree: The Evolution of Planning and Advising in Higher Education." https://d1hzkn4d3dn6lg.cloudfront.net/production/uploads/2019/03/TYT078_D2D18_Pt1_FINAL.pdf.

University of St. Augustine for Health Sciences. 2022. "The 2021 American Nursing Shortage: A Data Study." *University of St. Augustine for Health Sciences*, February 11, 2022. https://www.usa.edu/blog/nursing-shortage/.

U.S. Department of Education. 2022. "Report on the Condition of Education 2022." Institution of Education Sciences. https://nces.ed.gov/pubs2022/2022144.pdf.

U.S. Office of Personnel Management. 2019. "Reskilling Toolkit." President's Management Agenda. https://www.opm.gov/policy-data-oversight/workforce-restructuring/reshaping/accelerating-the-gears-of-transformation/reskilling-toolkit.pdf.

Vermeulen, Karla. 2021. *Generation Disaster Coming of Age Post-9/11*. New York: Oxford University Press.

VIA Institute on Character. 2018. *The VIA Survey of Character Strengths: United States Gen Z*. Data prepared by the VIA Institute on Character.

Vimal, Mourouguessine, Amol Rambhau Dongre, Anandabaskar Nishanthi, and Rajendrakumar Nivaratirao Kagne. 2021. "Student Support System for Medical Undergraduates: A Qualitative Exploration of Stakeholder Perspectives." *Journal of Education and Health Promotion*, *10*(150): 1–10. https://doi.org/10.4103/jehp.jehp_544_20.

Vogelsang, Markus, Katrin Rockenbauch, Hermann Wrigge, Wolfgang Heinke, and Gunther Hempel. 2018. "Medical Education for 'Generation Z': Everything Online?! – An Analysis of Internet-Based Media Use by Teacher in Medicine." *GMS Journal for Medical Education*, *35*(2): 1–10. https://doi.org/10.3205/zma001168.

Vuurberg, Gwendolyn, Julien A. M. Vos, L. H. Christoph, and Rien J. de Vos. 2019. "The Effectiveness of Interprofessional Classroom-Based Education in Medical Curricula: A Systematic Review." *Journal of Interprofessional Education & Practice*, *15*, 157–167. https://doi.org/10.1016/j.xjep.2019.01.007.

Waljee, Jennifer F, Vineet Chopra, and Sanjay Saint. 2020. "Mentoring Millenials." *JAMA*, *323*(17): 1716–1717. https://doi.org/10.1001/jama.2020.3085.

Walmsley, Laura, Melanie Fortune, and Allison Brown. 2018. "Experiential Interprofessional Education for Medical Students at a Regional Medical Campus." *Canadian Medical Education Journal*, *9*(1): e59–e67.

Wang, Yan, and Kevin B. Murphy. 2020. "A Comparison Study of NAEP-TEL and ICILS." U.S. Department of Education, Institute of Education Sciences, National Center for Education Statistics. https://nces.ed.gov/nationsreportcard/subject/tel/pdf/tel_icils_study.pdf.

Weinberg, Frankie J. 2019. "How and When Is Role Modeling Effective? The Influence of Mentee Professional Identity on Mentoring Dynamics and Personal Learning Outcomes." *Group & Organizational Management*, *44*(2): 425–477. https://doi.org/10.1177/1059601119838689.

Welch, Beth E., Sally A. Arif, Timothy J. Bloom, Alex N. Isaacs, Kirstin K. Janke, Jessica L. Johnson, Lindsey E. Moseley, and Libby J. Ross. 2020. "Report of the 2019–2020 AACP Student Affairs Standing Committee." *American Journal of Pharmaceutical Education*, *84*(10): Article 8198. https://doi.org/10.5688/ajpe8198.

WHO Study Group on Multiprofessional Education of Health Personnel: The Team Approach and World Health Organization. 1988. "Learning Together to Work Together for Health: Report of a WHO Study Group on Multiprofessional Education of Health Personnel: The Team Approach [meeting held in Geneva from 12 to 16 October 1987]." World Health Organization. https://apps.who.int/iris/handle/10665/37411; https://apps.who.int/iris/handle/10665/41063.

Wilbur, Kirsten, Cyndy Snyder, Alison C. Essary, Swapna Reddy, Kristen K. Will, and Mary Saxton. 2020. "Developing Workforce Diversity in the Health Professions: A Social Justice Perspective." *Health Professions Education*, *6*(2): 222–229. https://doi.org/10.1016/j.hpe.2020.01.002.

Wilkins, Emily B. 2021. "Fostering Professional Identity Formation in Generation Z Health Sciences Students." In *Cultivating Professional Identity Formation in the Health Sciences*, edited by Channing R. Ford, Lindsey E. Moseley, and Kimberly B. Garza. New Directions in Teaching and Learning, *2021*(168): 29–36. https://doi.org/10.1002/tl.20465.

Will, Kristen K., Melissa L. Johnson, and Gerri Lamb. 2019. "Team-Based Care and Patient Satisfaction in the Hospital Setting: A Systematic Review." *Journal of Patient-Centered Research and Reviews*, *6*(2): 158–171. https://doi.org/10.17294/2330-0698.1695.

Wingard, Jason. 2022. *The College Devaluation Crisis: Market Disruption, Diminishing ROI, and an Alternative Future of Learning*. Stanford, CA: Stanford Business Books, an imprint of Stanford University Press.

World Health Organization. 2010. "Framework for Action on Interprofessional Education and Collaborative Practice." Geneva: World Health Organization. https://apps.who.int/iris/handle/10665/70185.

World Health Organization. 2021. "What Is Patient Safety?" *Integrated Health Services, World Health Organization*. https://www.who.int/teams/integrated-health-services/patient-safety/about.

Yardley, Sarah, Pim W. Teunissen, and Tim Dornan. 2012. "Experiential Learning: Transforming Theory into Practice." *Medical Teacher*, *34*(2): 161–164. https://doi.org/10.3109/0142159X.2012.643264.

Yokotan, Mituse. 2011. "Recovering from Loss: A Qualitative Study Examining Student Loss While in Medical School." PhD diss, University of California, Los Angeles.

Young, Meredith E., Aliki Thomas, Stuart Lubarsky, David Gordon, Larry D. Gruppen, Joseph Rencic, Tiffany Ballard et al. 2020. "Mapping Clinical Reasoning Literature across the Health Professions: A Scoping Review." *BMC Medical Education*, *20*(1): 1–11. https://doi.org/10.1186/s12909-020-02012-9.

Zarra, Ernie J. 2017. *The Entitled Generation: Helping Teachers Teach and Reach the Minds and Hearts of Generation Z*. Lanham, MD: Rowman & Littlefield.

Zhang, Xiaoming, Daniel Lin, Hugh Pforsich, and Vernon W. Lin. 2010. "Physician Workforce in the United States of America: Forecasting Nationwide Shortages." *Human Resources for Health*, *18*(8). https://doi.org/10.1186/s12960-020-0448-3.

Index

About the Authors

Channing R. Ford, PhD, MPA, MA[2] is the dean of the graduate school and an assistant professor in the College of Education and Professional Studies at Jacksonville State University. She is responsible for the academic integrity and rigor of graduate and doctoral education and serves as the chair of the University's Graduate Curriculum Committee. Dr. Ford has authored over 30 peer-reviewed articles and book chapters. She conducts educational research in health professions education, scholarship of teaching and learning, assessment best practices, curricular development, deliberate practice, interprofessional education, professional identity formation, peer coaching, and mentoring.

Kimberly B. Garza, PharmD, MBA, PhD is an associate professor and graduate program officer in the Auburn University (AU) Harrison College of Pharmacy's Department of Health Outcomes Research and Policy. She also serves as a faculty fellow for the Biggio Center for the Enhancement of Teaching and Learning. Dr. Garza has authored over 60 peer-reviewed articles and book chapters. She also conducts educational research in the following areas: deliberate practice, empathy-building activities, curricular development, professional identity formation, peer coaching, and mentoring.

Lindsey E. Moseley, PharmD, PhD, MEd is a curricular coordinator at the Harrison College of Pharmacy at Auburn University. She oversees the implementation of coursework and assessments for all required courses in the first year of the highly integrated doctor of pharmacy (PharmD) curriculum. Dr. Moseley has a passion for advancing educational research in health professions. Her areas of study include professional identity formation, teaching and learning in pharmacy education, innovative curricula, and qualitative research.

Emily B. Wilkins, PhD, is the director for assessment and planning for the Division of Student Development at the University of Dayton. Dr. Wilkins serves as a first year seminar instructor and academic advisor for discovering students within the College of Arts and Sciences. She holds a doctorate in administration of higher education from Auburn University, with earned graduate certificates in college and university teaching, and program evaluation. Dr. Wilkins currently serves as a board member for the NASPA (Student Affairs Administrators in Higher Education) Center for Women. She has authored and co-authored peer reviewed publications in the areas of professional identity development, scholarship of teaching and learning, health professions education, generation theory, and gender issues for women in STEM.